PRACTICAL
PHARMACOGNOSY

PRACTICAL
PHARMACOGNOSY

By

Professor Rasheeduz Zafar
M. Pharm., Ph.D.
Dean Faculty of Pharmacy
Head of the Dept. of Pharmacognosy Phytochemistry
Faculty of Pharmacy
Hamdard University
New Delhi

and

Neerja Gandhi
M. Pharm.
Hamdard University
New Delhi

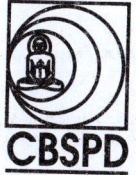

CBSPD

CBS Publishers & Distributors Pvt Ltd

New Delhi • Bengaluru • Chennai • Kochi • Kolkata • Lucknow • Mumbai
Hyderabad • Jharkhand • Nagpur • Patna • Pune • Uttarakhand

Practical Pharmacognosy

ISBN: 978-81-239-0271-5

Copyright © Authors & Publishers

First Edition: 1994

Reprint: 2000, 2004, 2005, 2006, 2007, 2009, 2013, 2017, 2018, 2019, 2020, 2023, 2024

Published by Satish Kumar Jain and Produced by Varun Jain for

CBS Publishers & Distributors Pvt Ltd

4819/XI Prahlad Street, 24 Ansari Road, Daryaganj, New Delhi 110 002, India.4819/XI Prahlad Street, 24 Ansari Road, Daryaganj, New Delhi 110 002, India.

Ph: 23289259, 23266861   Website: www.cbspd.com
e-mail: delhi@cbspd.com

Corporate Office: 204 FIE, Industrial Area, Patparganj, Delhi 110 092

Ph: 011-4934 4934   Fax: 011-4934 4935   e-mail: publishing@cbspd.com;
publicity@cbspd.com

Branches

- **Bengaluru:** Seema House 2975, 17th Cross, K.R. Road, Banasankari 2nd Stage, Bengaluru 560 070, Karnataka
  Ph: +91-80-26771678/79   Fax: +91-80-26771680   e-mail: bangalore@cbspd.com
- **Chennai:** 7, Subbaraya Street, Shenoy Nagar, Chennai 600 030, Tamil Nadu, India
  Ph: +91-44-26680620/26681266   Fax: +91-44-42032115   e-mail: chennai@cbspd.com
- **Kochi:** 42/1325, 1326, Power House Road, Opp KSEB, Power House, Ernakulam 682 018, Kochi, Kerala, India
  Ph: +91-484-4059061-65, 67   Fax: +91-484-4059065   e-mail: kochi@cbspd.com
- **Kolkata:** 147, Hind Ceramics Compound, 1st Floor, Nilgunj Road, Belghoria, Kolkata-700056, West Bengal, India
  Ph: +033-25633055, 033-25633056   e-mail: kolkata@cbspd.com
- **Lucknow:** Basement, Khushnuma Complex, 7 Meerubai Marg (Behind Jawahar Bhawan), Lucknow-226001, UP, India
  Ph: +91-522-4000032   e-mail: tiwari.lucknow@cbspd.com
- **Mumbai:** PWD Shed, Gala no 25/26, Ramchandra Bhatt Marg, Next to JJ Hospital Gate no. 2, Opp. Union Bank of India Noorbaug, Mumbai-400009, Maharashtra, India
  Ph: 022-66661880/89   e-mail: mumbai@cbspd.com

Representatives

• **Hyderabad**	0-9885175004	• **Jharkhand**	0-9811541605	• **Nagpur**	0-8692091830
• **Patna**	0-9334159340	• **Pune**	0-9664372571	• **Uttarakhand**	0-9716462459

Printed at: Glorious Printers, Jhilmil Industrial Area, Delhi, India

PREFACE

Diseases were known to man since the origin of human race, the causes of which were not known. They were assumed to be evil spirits. So people tried to treat the diseases with plants easily available to them. Value of medicinal plants started accumulating and our ancestors preserved it in literature. Regveda (4500-1600 B.C.) appears to be the oldest book giving information about medicinal plants. After Rigveda work of Susruta (in surgery) and Charaka (in medicine) appeared as medical literature. In all the old texts description of plants has been given preference to other characteristics.

The identification of crude drugs is an important aspect of the curriculum of Pharmacognosy and related branches. It is because of the fact that unless the true identity of drug is not established by studying the morphological characters, other characteristics remain less significant Visual observation is the sole source of information as we do not use any instrument or apparatus and thus error is minimised.

Students must be well acquainted with the studies of external characters of crude drugs including organoleptic tests.

The present book contains practical details as prescribed in the Education Regulation 1991 of Pharmacy Council of India. Description and diagrams are informative and students can understand the text and diagrams in correct prospectives. Every detail in the book is included with a view to help students so that they can express themselves correctly and fluently in practicals.

The authors are hopeful that the book will fulfill the expectation of diploma as well as degree studens of pharmacy. We have made all efforts to make it an ideal book, however we shall look forward to valuable suggestions for the improvement of the book.

Acknowledgement : We are thankful to Mr. Sanjay Gandhi for this assistance in sketching the drawings and useful suggestions in arranging the diagrams and text. We are also thankful to Janab Hkm. Abdul Hameed, Chancellor, Jamia Hamdard, New Delhi and to Mr. Abdul Mueed for their encouragement.

Rasheeduz Zafar
Neerja Gandhi

CONTENTS

GENERAL NOTES ON PRACTICAL ASPECTS

Identification of various drugs by their morphological characters is an important aspect of pharmacognostical identification of drugs. It includes morphology (study of the form) along with morphography (description of the form) for the specimens of known crude drugs. Majority of the natural drugs are derived from the plants and part of plants where the active constituents are concentrated. The following are the basic groups under which the drugs come.

A. ORGANISED DRUGS

1. Leaf
2. Flower or Bud
3. Fruit
4. Seed
5. Bark
6. Wood
7. Herb or aerial parts
8. Underground organs like roots and rhizomes

B. UNORGANISED DRUGS

1. Gum
2. Resins
3. Extract and juices

Leaves are broadly classified as simple leaves and compound leaves. In simple leaf is having one lamina (which may be undivided or lobed) bears axillay bud in the axil e.g. vasaka, digitatis, castor (lobed). Compound leaves leaf blade is divided into several segments called e.g. leaflets of senna, acacia.

1. DESCRIPTION OF LEAFY DRUG

Leaves are of two types

Leaf is flatted lateral outgrowth of stem. Its description can be given by using various terms as :

1. *Dimension* : Length and breadth
2. *Attachment* : Leaf stalk or petiole present or absent (sessile)
3. *Lamina* : It is the flat part of leaf. It may be thick or thin.
4. *Stipules* : Outgrowth at the base of leaf. If it is present leaf is stipulated leaf, if absent ex-stipulated. It may be foliaceous or spiny
5. *LeafLamina shape* : Varies in different types of leaves. It may be linear, lanceolate, ovate to obovate

Note : For dry samples the shape can be determined by soaking in warm water.

Leaf margin : The margin may be entire, crenate, serrate, dentate or sinuate.

Leaf apex : The tip of lamina may be of different types like acute, acuminate obtuse, emarginate.

Leaf base : Lower part of lamina may be symmetrical or assymetrical.

Leaf texture : The drug may be found as whole or broken form and may be described as shrivelled, brittle, papery, fleshy or coriaceous.

Venation : It is the arrangement of veins on the lamina It may be reticulate or parallel.

Leaf surface : It may the glabrous (free form hair & smooth), rough, hairy, glaucous or pubescent.

Phyllotaxy : Arrangement of leaves, on the stem may be alternate, opposite, whorled or opposite decussate (e.g. vinca).

Various modifications found in leaves are leaf tendril (wiry structure coiled), leaf spine (aloe), scale leaves (ginger, garlic, onion).

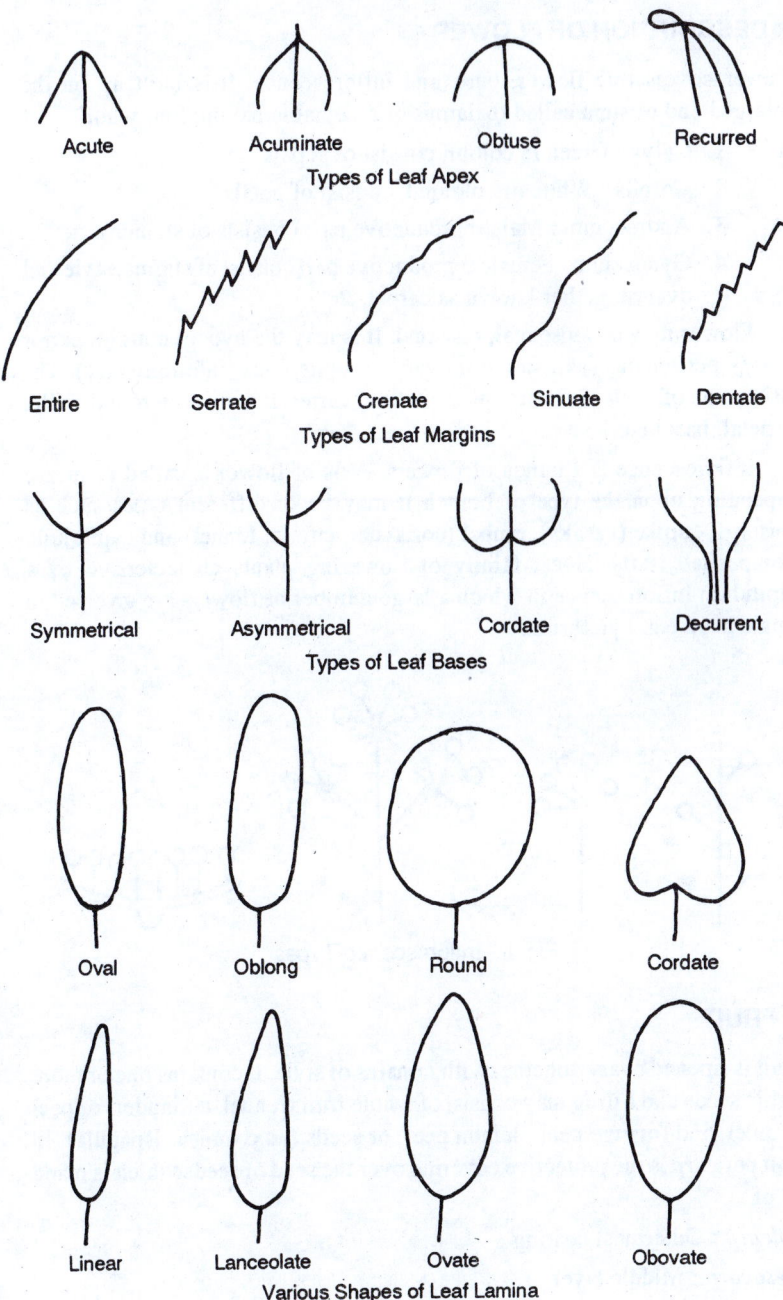

Acute   Acuminate   Obtuse   Recurred

Types of Leaf Apex

Entire   Serrate   Crenate   Sinuate   Dentate

Types of Leaf Margins

Symmetrical   Asymmetrical   Cordate   Decurrent

Types of Leaf Bases

Oval   Oblong   Round   Cordate

Linear   Lanceolate   Ovate   Obovate

Various Shapes of Leaf Lamina

Fig. I. Leaf base margin

2. DESCRIPTION OF FLOWER

Flower covers true flower, buds and inflorescence. It is built up on the enlarged end of stem called thalamus or receptable having four whorls.

1. Calyx : Green in colour, consist of sepals
2. Corolla : White or coloured, consist of petals
3. Androecium : Male reproductive part consists of stamens
4. Gynoecium : Female reproductive part consist of stigma, style and ovary together known as carpel.

Flower may be unisexual, bisexual. It is may the hypogynous (superior ovary), perigynous (half superior ovary) or epigynous (inferior ovary). The discription of ovules in ovary (placentation) varies. It may be marginal, axile, parietal, basal etc.

Inflorescence is a bunch of flowers. Axis of flower is called peduncle depending upon the type of branch It may be of different types such as mustard, spike (vasaka), umbel (coriander, cumin, fennel) and capitulum. Compositae is the lagest family of flowering plants characterised by a capitulum inflorescence in which a large number of flowers are grouped in single head e.g. pyrethrum.

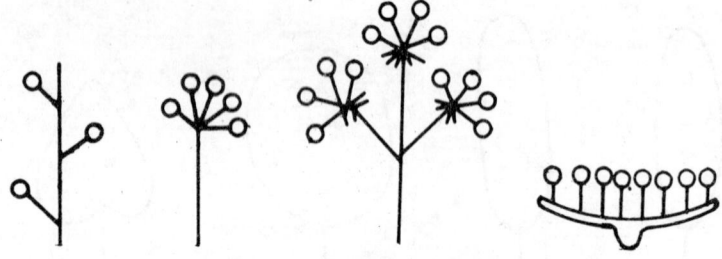

Fig. II. Inflorescence Types

3. FRUIT

Fruit is ripened ovary together with remains of style. It contains one or more fertile seeds and a drug may consist of whole fruit (fennel, coriander) or peel or outer rind (orange peel , lemon peel) or seeds (nuxvomica, Ispagula). In fruit pericarp is the protective covering over the seed or seeds which is made up of :

Epicarp : Outermost coating

Mesocarp : Middle layer

Endocarp : Innermost layer

Fruits may be simple (developed from single carpel) or aggregate (formed from many carpels). They may be further dry (coriander, fennel) or fleshy (orange, lemon).

Dry fruits may be dehiscent (cardamom) indehiscent (fennel). Schizocarp is a special type of indehiscent fruit in which cremocarp of umbelliferae are important fruits. The cremocarp consist of two carpels each containing one seed derived from inferior ovary. The two halves of the cremocarp are called mericarps. Each mericarp has flat surface called commisural surface and rounded surface called dorsal surface. Carpophore is the suture like structure from which the mericarps break loose. Each mericarp usually has the prominent primary ridges and the non-prominent secondary ridges in between the primary ridges. At the apex remains of style and calyx form stylopod.

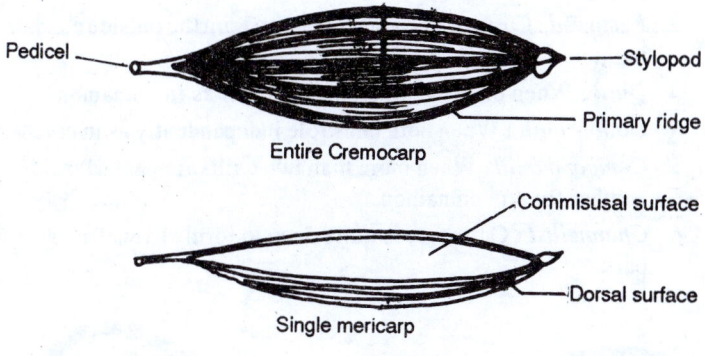

Fig. III. Cremocarp

4. SEEDS

Seed is a fertilised ovule. The seeds are characterised by the presence of three parts namely seed coat, embryo, endosperm. Seed coat may be thick (dicot) or thin (monocot). Embryo contains the apical meristem for radicle (root apex), plumule (shoot apex) and one or two cotyledons.

Endosperm is the nutritive tissue nourishing the embryo. The seeds are classed as endospermic (exalbuminous) for e.g. Colchicum. Non endospermic (exalbuminous) for e.g cotton or perispermic for e.g. nutmeg, pepper. Other terms used with the seeds are :

Hilum : It is point of attachment of seed to its stalk

Micropyle : It is minute opening for the absorption of water.

Raphe : Longitudinal marking of adherent stalk.

Chalaza : Basal portion of ovule.

Aril : Succulent growth covering the entire seed for e.g. nutmeg.

Arillode : Outgrowth from micropyle covering the seed such as in cardamom.

Strophiole : It is the enlarged funicle for e.g. colchicum.

Hair : Sometimes present as in cotton.

5. DESCRIPTION OF BARK

Commercially 'bark' includes all those tissues external to cambium in a mature, secondarily thickened stem. The shape of bark varies and it depends upon the type of incision given in removing them from the tree. When it is removed from large trees it is usually flat but becomes curved when removed from smaller branching in drying. Curling on drying is due to unequal shrinkage of various layers. Special terms are used to describe them.

1. *Curved :* When slightly curved
2. *Recurved* : Curved such that concavity is on the outside e.g. kurchi bark.
3. *Quill* : When one edge overlaps the other as in cinnamon
4. *Double quill* : When both ends role independently as in cinchona.
5. *Compond quill* : When more than two quills are packed inside one aonther for e.g. cinnamon.
6. *Channelled* : Curvature is quite deep to form channel as in cassia bark.

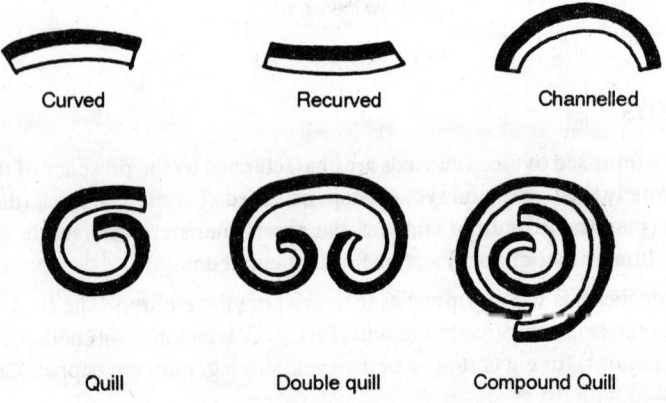

Curved   Recurved   Channelled

Quill   Double quill   Compound Quill

Fig. IV. Types of Bark

Some barks are naturally smooth in appearance while some are rough, may become wrinkled or exfoliate. Sometimes epiphytes, lichens or mosses may appear on the surface. Lichens give silvery grey appearance while mosses are green.

Fracture of bark is an important feature and it is the appearance of exposed surface when the bark is broken transversely. It is of following types:

Short : When fractured surface is smooth

Granular : Surface show rounded protuberances

Splintery : Surface show projecting points

Fibrous : When threads extend from broken regions.

Laminated : Fractured region breaks into tangentially arranged layers.

Wood

Wood is the tissue laying inside the cambium and consist mainly of xylem with small amount of other types of cells e.g. Quassia wood.

6. HERB OR AERIAL ORGANS

Herb consist of entire aerial parts of young plant composed of leaves, stems, flowers and young fruits so description of each part must be explained.

7. UNDERGROUND ORGANS

This includes roots and rhizomes. Rhizome resembles the root superficially and its internal arrangement bears the structure of stem. But they can be distinguished from the roots. Rhizomes develop from the part of mature plant other than the radicle.

Root has no central pith, scale leaves or axillary bud and it only develops from the radicle of germinating seedling. The underground modifications of stem are tuber (for e.g. aconite), bulb (scilla, garlic) and corm (colchicum) various terms used for describing root or rhizome are peeled, sliced, or whole. The shape may be described in terms of straight, branching, cylindrical, conical or tortous. Scale leaves, root scars or lenticles may be present and fracture may be short, fibrous splintery or starchy.

B. DESCRIPTION FOR UNORGANISED DRUGS

Unorganised drugs form the acellular products. They may the solid or liquid (fixed essental oils). For describing the solid drugs size, shape of pieces, surface appearance (dull, smooth or cracked), fracture (short, rough) and texture (hard, brittle or crumbling).

Various types of unorganised drugs include the following categores.

Gums : Exudates obtained by making incision to bark. Some exudes slowly dry into ovoid tears (acacia) and some exudes rapidly under pressure for e.g. tragacanth, acacia.

Resins : They are heterogenous group of materials. They are brittle amorphus solids, when melted form adhesive liquids. They may occur with essential oils as oleo resins (for e.g. colophony) with gums in gum resins (e.g. myrrh) and as solutions in liquid esters as in balsams (e.g. balasm of tolu).

Dried extracts and juices : They form number of important products e.g. Aloe as the dried juice obtained from cut leaves of various species of Aloe, Catechu in the dried aqueous extract obtained from certain tannin containing plants. Opium is the dried latex from the capsule of poppy.

2
LAXATIVES

1. ALOES

OFFICIAL SOURCE

The residue obtained by evaporating to dryness the liquid which drains from the leaves cut from various species of Aloe, is known in commerce as cape or curacao (or Barbadoes) aloes. The important species are : *Aloe ferox,* yielding Cape Aloes, *Aloe vera* Linn var *officinalis* (Forsk) Baker, yielding Indian and Curacao Aloes, *Aloe perryi* Baker, giving Socotrine Aloes and Zanzibar Aloes,

Family : Liliaceae.

PHYSICAL CHARACTERISTICS

Two forms of aloes are available according to its method of preparation:

1. **Hepatic, livery or opaque :** This form is produced by slow evaporation of the aloetic juice, a process which is favourable to crystallzation of one of its constituents, namely barbaloin. Under the microscope this substance may be seen in minute crystals and their presence renders this form of aloes opaque to the eye.

2. **Vitrous, glassy, or transparent :** This form is produced by rapid evaporation of the aloetic juice at or near to its boilng points a process unfavourable to crystallization of the barbaloin. As a consequence this form is free from embeded crystals, and appears transparent and glassy.

The general comparative characters, given below have reference to typical specimens but in commerce the drug exhibits considera. variation.

Physical Charactersitics of Different Aloes

	Curacao	Socotrine	Zanzibur	Cape
Form	Unusally opaque some what translucent	Opaque	Opaque	Transparent & glassy
Colour	Reddish brown to chocolate brown	Dark brown	Liver colour	Dark brown or greenish brown
Fracture	Smooth, even and wax like	Porous (due to vesicles)	Fairly smooth porous	Smooth even & glassy
Odour	Strong & unpleasent	Slight & disagreeable	Pleasent some times myrrh like	Unpleasent peculiar & distinct from others
Taste	Disagreeably bitter taste	Disagreeably bitter taste	Disagreeably bitter taste	Disagreebly bitter taste

CHEMICAL TESTS

Brontrager's test: Boil 0.1 g of the powdered drug with 5 ml of 10% sulphuric acid for 2 minutes. Filter while hot, cool the filtrate & shake gently with equal volume of benzene. Allow the benzene layer to separate completely from the lower layer and by means of a teal pipette and transfer the benzene layer to a clean test tube. Add about half its volume of aqueous solution of ammonia (10%). Shake gently and allow the layer to separate. The lower ammonical layer will acquire red pink colour due to the presence of free anthraquinones.

Modified Borntrager's test : The C-glycosides of anthraquinones requires more drastic conditions for hydrolysis and thus a modification of the above test is to use ferric chloride and hydrochloric acid to effect oxidative hydrolysis. 0.1 g of the drug 5 ml dil, hydrochloric acid and 5 ml of 5% solution of ferric chloride are boiled for 5 minutes, cool the solution and filter. This filterate is shaken with benzene. Separate the benzene layer and add an equal volume of dilute solution of ammonia. The ammonical layer shows pink colour.

Borax test : Boil 0.5 g of the drug with 50 ml water, add 0.5 g of kieselguhr, stir it well and filter through filter paper. The filtrate is divided into two parts. With one part of the filtrate perform borax test and the second part is kept for the Bromine test. To the filtrate add 0.2 g of borax and heat, out of this solution take about 10 drops and dilute to 10 ml in a test tube and see against ordinary day light. Green flourescence is observed due to the presence of aloe-emodin.

Bromine test : To the solution of aloe prepared in the above test add equal volume of bromine solution. Bulky yellow precipitates are immediately formed due to the formation of *tetrabromaloin.*

Cupraloin test : To dilute aqueous solution of aloe add a drop of copper sulphate solution. Bright yellow colour is obtained which changes to purple on addition of 2 ml of saturated solution of sodium chloride. This colour persists on addition of 4 ml of 90% alcohol. This test is due to the presence of iso-barbaloin and is strongly positive with Scotorine aloe due to the presence of isobarbaloin.

Nitrous acid test : To 5 ml of aqueous solution of aloe, add a few small crystals of sodium nitrite and 2-3 drops of dilute acetic acid. Pink or purple colour is obtained.

2. RHUBARB

The drug consists of peeled and dried rhizomes and roots of *Rheum officinale* Baillon and other species of Rheum except *Rheum rhaponticum* L The drug is also known as Chinese rhubarb. Indian rhubarb is obtained from the roots and rhizomes of *R. emodi* wall, *R. webianum* and other species.

Family : Polygonaceae

PHYSICAL CHARACTERS

Chinese rhubarbs 'Round' (prepared from smaller rhizome)

1. *Form and Size* : Cylindrical, barrel shaped or conical pieces 5-12 cm. long; 3-8 cm. is diameter.
2. *Surface characters* : Smooth, pale brown to reddish brown and mottled. The mottled appearance is seen to be due to small groups of reddish-brown tissues (medullary ray) distributed in whitish tissue, the latter forming interlacing white lines. Occasionally "star-spots" and small reddish patches of bark. Often perforated with a hole about 3-4 mm in diameter, which sometimes contains a portion of the rope on which of the rhizone was strung for the purpose of drying.
3. *Texture* : Compact, firm and diffuse.
4. *Fracture* : Granular and uneven, the broken surface appearing distinctly mottled, an appearance refered to as the "nutmeg" fracture. Finest quality has a bright pink tinge on the freshly fractured surface.

CHINESE RHUBARB "FLATS"

It is Prepared by Longitudinally slicing the Large Rhizoms

1. *Form and size* : Plano-convex, upto 15 cm in length and 5 cm in thickness.
2. *Surface characters* : As above, star-spots being particularly numerous on the flat inner surface.

INDIAN RHUBARB

1. *Form and size* : It occurs in much shrunken cylindrical or irregular pieces. Light in weight soft and easily cut.
2. *Surface character* : It is darker (Yellow brown) in colour than chinese rhubarb.
3. *Odour* : Faint characteristic
4. *Taste* : Bitter and astringent.

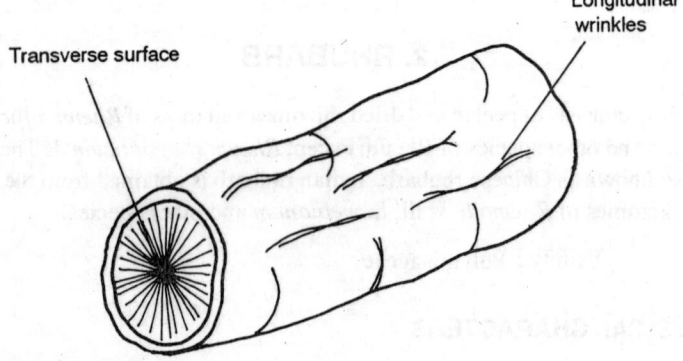

Transverse surface

Longitudinal wrinkles

Fig. 1. Rhubarb

CHEMICAL TEST

1. Bontrager's and its modified tests described under aloe are positive due to the presence of anthraquinone glycosides.
2. Powered rhubarb when treated with 5 percent potassium hydroxide gives a blood red colour.
3. Extract 0.5 g of the drug with 10 ml of 45% alcohol by macerating for 20 minutes, filter and place a drop of the filtrate on a piece of filter paper and examine under ultra violet light. No blue colour should appear in the *genuine* official drug. But if the blue colour appears in this test then the drug is adultrated with *rhaphontic* rhubarb which gives this blue colour due to the presence of a glycoside rhaponticin which is a stilbene derivative. This glycoside is not present in any other rhubarb species which are used as drug.

3. CASTOR OIL

Castor oil is a fixed oil obtained from the seeds of *Ricinus communis*

Family : Euphorbiaceae

Physical and Chemical Characters

Medicinal castor oil is a colourless or pale yellow liquid, with a slight odour and faintly acrid taste. The oil is soluble in alcohol and this is an exceptional property which is lacking in all other fixed oils. It is miscible with all other organic solvents. The acid value of the oil should not be mare than 2 but it increases if the extraction is carelessly done or the damaged seeds are used for extracting oil. The oil is viscous having specific gravity 0.945-0.965, iodine value is 82-90 and saponification value 177-185.

TESTS

Some of the more important are given below solubility tests are best means of detecting adultration.

1. *Solubility in alcohol* : Other fixed oils are only slightly soluble in 90% alcohol at normal temperature, whereas castor oil is characterized by complete solublity in 2 parts of 90% alcohol. Castor oil gives a clear solution with an equal volume dehydrated alcohol.

2. *Partial solubility in light petroleum* : Most fixed oils mix in all proportions with light petroleum. Castor oil yields a clear liquid with half its own volume of light petroleum, but when more of the latter (to form twice the volume of the oil) is added the liquid becomes turbid, and on standing, separates into two layers.

3. *Weight per ml.* : This is the highest of any natural fixed oil.

4. *Optical rotation* : Fixed oil are usually optically inactive but not so with castor oil, because an asymmetric carbon atom is present in ricinoleic acid. The optical rotation must be not less than + 3.5 Hydnocarpus oil is also optically active.

5. It is miscible with hydrated alcohol and with glacial acetic acid.

4. ISPAGHULA

The drug consists of seeds of *Plantago ovata Forsk.*

Family : Plantaginaceae

Ispaghula husk consists of the epidermis separated from the seeds.

PHYSICAL CHARACTERS

Size : Length, 1.8-3.3 mm, width 1.0-1.7 mm

Shape : Ovate, boat shaped.

Dorsal surface : Convex, dull, opaque pinkish gray, a slight transverse constriction in the equatorial region, corresponding to the line of dehiscene of the capsule.

Ventral surface : A deep furrow, not quite reaching either end of the seed Hilum : central appearing as a red-brown, oval spot.

Odour : None

Taste : Mucilageneous

Weight : 100 seeds weight 0.15-0.19 g

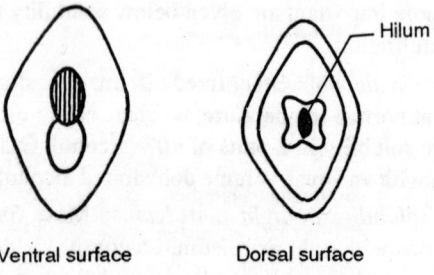

Ventral surface   Dorsal surface

Fig. 2. Ispaghula

Determination of Swelling Factor

1.0 g of the seeds are agitated gently and occasionally in a measuring cylinder filled upto 20 ml with water and allowed to stand 24 hours. The seeds swell and occupy not less than 12 ml.

5. SENNA

The drug consists of dried leaflets and pods of *Cassia angustifolia* Vahl (Tinnevelly senna) or *Cassia acutifolia* Delile (Alexendrian senna).

    Family : Leguminosae

Morphological Characters

Characters	Cassia angustifolia	Cassia acutifolia
1. Colour	Pale yellowish green, the yellow colour more pronounced on upper surface	Pale greyish green
2. Texture	Thin & some what flexible	Thin and brittle
3. Hairs	Scattered over both surfaces short usually pale & covered near the base	Some as in Tinnevelly senna. Numberous on Alexendrian senna
4. Taste	Mucilaginous	Mucilaginous
5. Odour	Faint, but distinctive	Faint, but distinctive
6. Size	2.5-5.0 cm long	2.0-4.0 cm long
7. Shape	Lanceolate, only slightly asymmetrical	Ovate lanceolate, conspicuously asymmetrical
8. Margin	Entire, flat	Entire, curved
9. Apex	Less acute and with a sharp spine	Acute with a sharp spine
10. Base	Somewhet asymmetrical	Conspicuously asymmetrical
11. Veins	Pinnate, distinct on the lower surface.	Pinnate

MORPHOLOGY OF THE PODS

The pods are unilocular, laterally flattened and dehiscing by both sutures. They are about 5 cm long and 2 cm broad having broad oblong shape, round apex and contain 5-8 seeds.

CHEMICAL TESTS

Borntrager's and modified Borntrager's test as given under aloe are positive due to the presence of anthraquinone derivatives.

T.S. OF LEAFLET

1. **Epidermis (upper and lower)** : Polygonal tulular cells having straight anticlinal walls. The inner periclinal wall contain mucilage and can be stained with ruthenium red. The epidermal trichomes are simple,

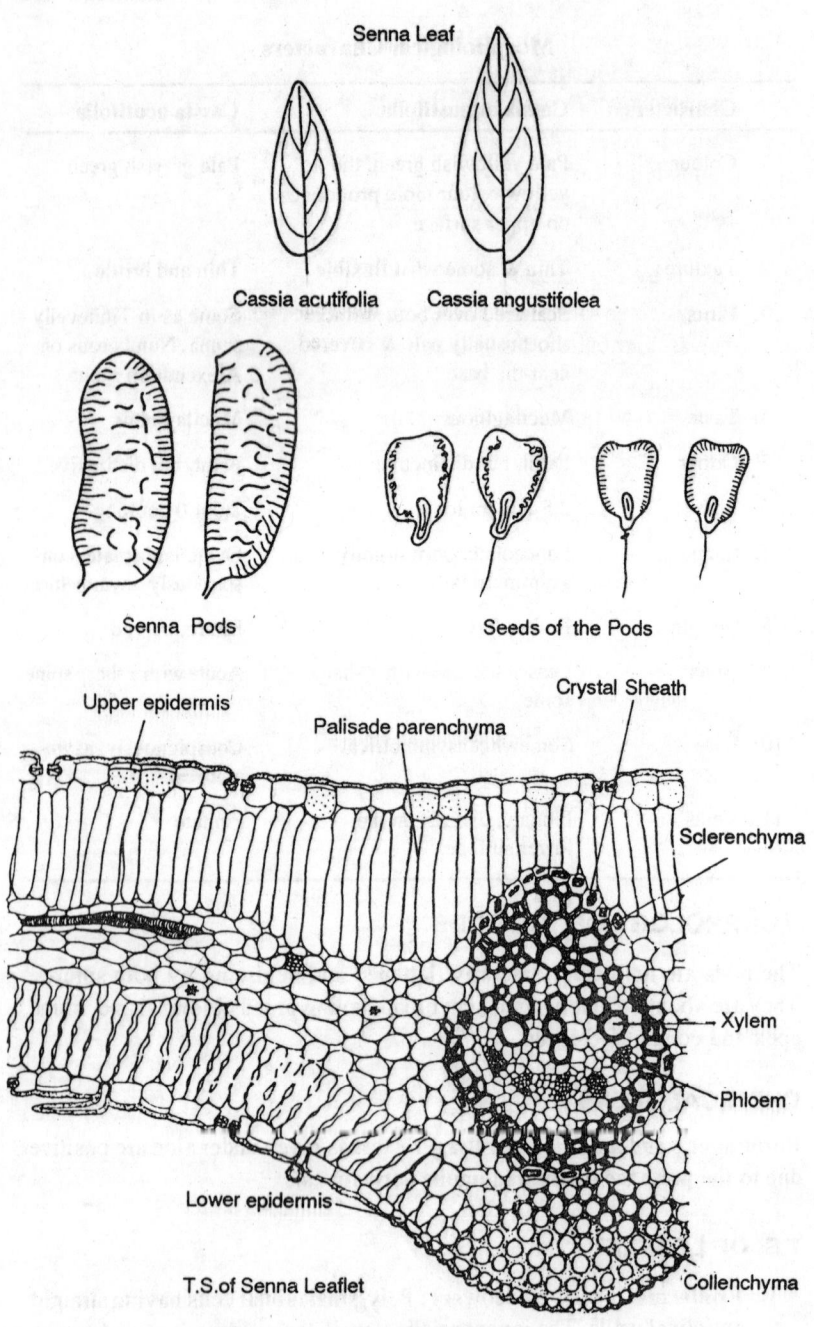

Senna Leaf

Cassia acutifolia   Cassia angustifolea

Senna Pods   Seeds of the Pods

Upper epidermis   Palisade parenchyma   Crystal Sheath

Sclerenchyma

Xylem

Phloem

Lower epidermis

T.S.of Senna Leaflet   Collenchyma

Fig. 3. Senna

covering, conical, thin walled with warty cuticle and are curved at the base. The stomata present are of paracytic type. (paracytic type of stomata can only be seen in the surface view of the epidermins).

2. **Palisade layer :** A single layer is present on upper and lower surface (isobilateral leaf)

3. **Spongy tissues :** Parenchymatous cell which are loosely arranged Clusture crystals of calcium oxalate are present in them. There are few vessels having special thickness.

4. **Midrib :** Shows collenchyma, sclerenchyma layer on both the sides of the vascular bundle consisting of xylem and phloem.

5. Prismatic Calcium oxalate crystals are present in crystal sheath which are also seen in powder of senna.

3

CARDIOTONICS

1. DIGITALIS

Digitalis (foxglove leaves) consists of dried leaves of *Digitalis purpurea* linn.
Family : Scrophulariaceae

Morphology

1. *Size* : 10 - 30 cm Long 4 - 10 cm wide
2. *Shape* : Broadly ovate to ovate lanceolate upper leaves and first year lower leaves are narrow.
3. *Margin* : Crenate or irregularly crenate serrate
4. *Apex* : Blunt or somewhat acute.
5. *Base* : Lamina narrows and forms a winged petiole. Lower leaves and first year leaves have longer petiole.
6. *Veins* : Midrib prominent, lateral viens leave at an acute angle, curve, and tend to run parallel to the margin. The lower veins pass into the winged petiole and join the midrib lower down.
7. *Colour* : Upper surface dull green (and wrinkled) under surface paler.
8. *Texture* : Brittle, upper surface less hairy, lower surface densely covered with trichomes.
9. *Taste* : Bitter
10. *Odour* : Scarcely perceptible

MORPHOLOGY OF DIGILATICS LANATA

1. *Size* : 25-30 cm long, 4-5 cm wide
2. *Shape* : Linear, lanceolate sessile leaves

3. *Margin* : Entire

4. *Apex* : Acuminate

5. *Base* : Basal half ciliate with long uniseriate trichomes; otherwise the leaf is glabrous.

6. *Veins* : The main veins are few, they leave into midrib at a very acute angle and travel for some distance towards the apex while the smaller branches are inconspicuous, showing a parallel vention.

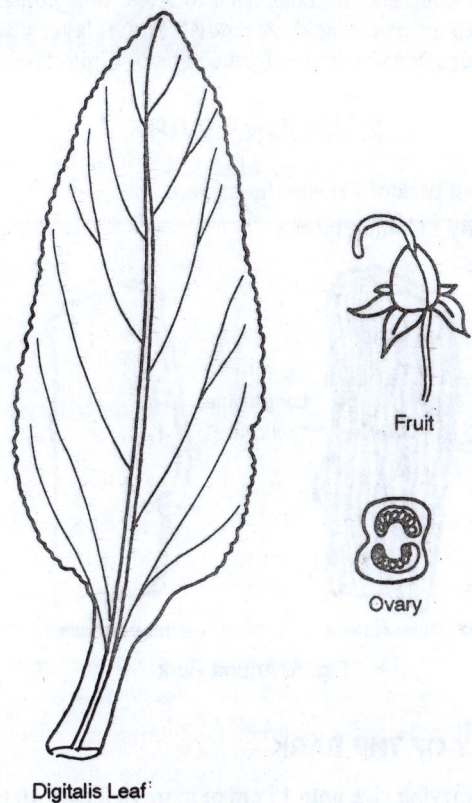

Fruit

Ovary

Digitalis Leaf

Fig. 4. Digitalis Leaf

CHEMICAL TESTS

1. **Baljet test** : A thick section of the leaf with sodium picrate reagent shows yellow to orange colour.

2. **Legal test** : Dissolve the glycoside (.1 g) in pyridine (2 ml) and sodium

nitroprusside solution (2 ml) and make alkaline with sodium hydroxide solution. It shows pink to red colour.

3. **Killer-Kiliani test for deoxy sugars :** Boil about 1g of the powered drug with 70% alcohol for 3 minutes, filter and to the filtrate add 5 ml water and 0.5 ml of strong solution of lead acetate, shake well and filter. The clear filtrate in extracted with equal volume of chloroform and chloroform layer is evaporated. The residue is dissolved in 3 ml of glacial acetic acid and to this two drops of ferric chloride solution are added. The contents are transferred to a test tube containing 2 ml of concentrated sulphuric acid. A reddish brown layer acquiring bluish green colour after standing is formed due to digitoxose.

2. ARJUNA BARK

Arjuna is the dried bark of *Terminalia arjuna*.

    Family : Combretaceae

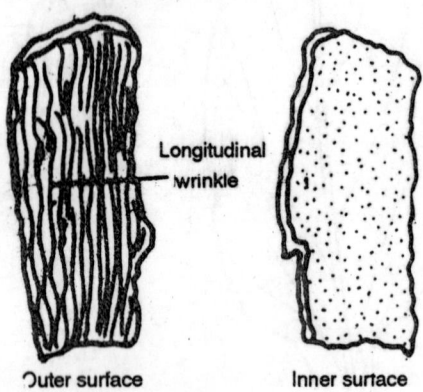

Fig. 5. Arjuna Bark

MORPHOLOGY OF THE BARK

Size : Pieces of varying size upto 15 cm or more in length 10 cm or more in breadth and 3 mm to 1 cm thick.

Shape : Flat or slightly curved.

Outer surface : Smooth and grey, coloured

Inner surface : Finely striated, brown

Fracture : Short revealing stratified nature of the bark.

Odour : None

Taste : Astringent

CHEMICAL TESTS

The cynogenetic glycocides present in the drug may be identified by the following tests which depend on the liberation of volatile hydrocyanic acid.

1. **Grignard reaction or sodium picrate test :** Dip a slip of while filter paper in 1% aqueous solution of picric acid drain it and dip in a 10% sodium carbonate solution and drain again, bruise or powder the drug, moisten it with water and put into a conical flask. Trap the sodium paper on the neck of the flask with cork because of volatile hydrocynic acid, the paper will become brick red or maroon coloured.

2. With 3% aqueous solution of mercurous nitrate reduction to metallic mercury take place. This test can be used as localisation test.

3. **Fluorescence Test :** Arjuna bark extract (10%) in ether shows a pinkish white and petroleum ether extract shows bright pinkish red fluorescence.

CARMINATIVES AND G.I. REGULATORS

1. CORIANDER

Coriander is the dried ripe fruit obtained from *Coriandrum sativum*.

Family : Umbelliferae

Morphological characters

General appearance : Entire cremocarp with pedicel

Size : 3 to 4 mm in diameter

Shape : Subspherical

Surface : A short stylopod with 5 small calyx teeth present at apex. Ten inconspicuous wavy primary ridges present.

Colour : Yellowish brown

Odour : Aromatic

Taste : Spicy, aromatic

T.S. OF CORIANDER

The cremocarp is divided into two mericarps. T.S. of mericarp show two prominent surfaces dorsal and commisural. It has 5 less prominent primary ridges and 4 prominent secondary ridges. In the ripe fruit dorsal surface has no vittae Mericarp show the following structures in T.S.

Epidermis of the pericarp is composed of polygonal tabular cells. Prism crystal of calcium oxalate are present occassionally.

Mesocarp : It is composed of outer and inner layer of parenchyma and in between lignified sclerenchymatous cells in sinous rows. They tend to be

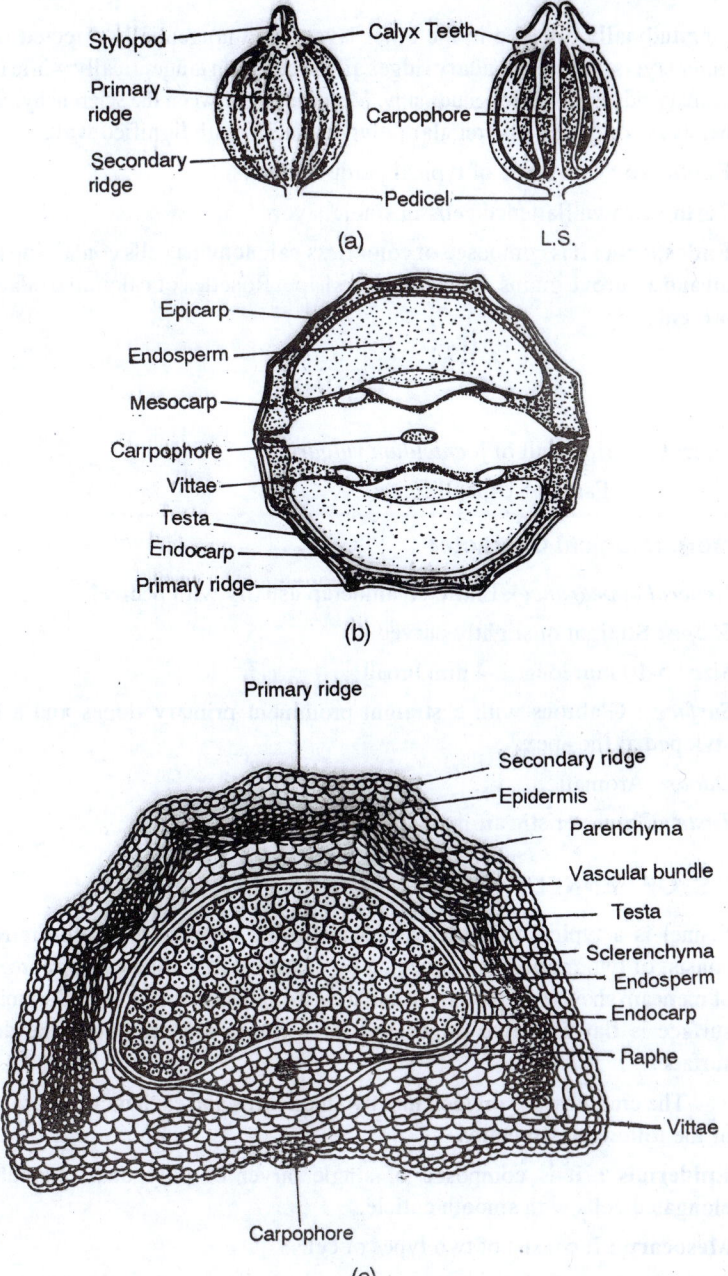

Fig. 6. Coriander

longitudinally directed in the outer layers, and tangentially directed in the inner layers. In the secondary ridges all the cells run tangentically while in the primary ridges all run longitudinally. Mesocarp in between the sclerenchymatous bands is composed of irregular polygonal cells with lignified walls.

Endocarp : It is made of typical parquetry cells.

Testa : Brown flattened cells in single layer.

Endosperm : It is composed of colourless parenchyma cells containing fixed oil and aleurone grains. It is curved in shape. Rosettes of calcium oxalate are present.

2. FENNEL

Fennel is a ripe fruit of *foeniculum vulgare*
           Family : Umbelliferae

Morphological Character

General appearance : Entire creamocrap usually with pedicel

Shape : Straight or slightly curved

Size : 5-10 mm long. 2-4 mm broad

Surface : Glabrous with 5 straight prominent primary ridges and a bifid stylopod at the apex.

Odour : Aromatic

Taste : Characteristic aromatic taste.

T.S. OF FENNEL

Fennel is a typical umbelliferous fruit called cremocarp. Each cremocrp consist of two mericarps connected by central stalk called carpophore. T.S. of mericarp shows two prominent surfaces. Commisural and dorsal. Commisural surface is flat with two ridges and three ridges are present in the dorsal surface. .

   The cremocarp is divided into two mericarps and each mericarp consists of the following structures.

Epidermis : It is composed of single laryer of polygonal tangentially elongated cells with smooth cuticle.

Mesocarp : It consist of two types of cells.

Reticulate lignified parenchyma is present surrounding the bicollateral vascular bundles while the other type is made up of ordinary polyhedral cells.

Vittae : Four yellowish brown elliptical vittae are present on the dorsal surface between the ridges and two on the commisural surface.

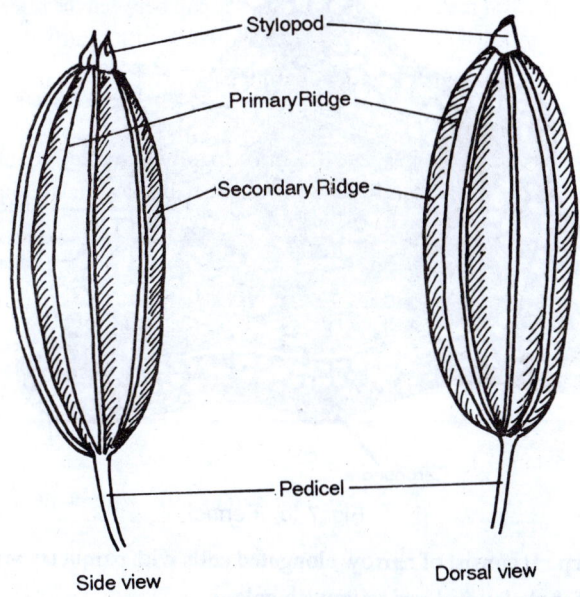

Fig. 7(a) Fennel

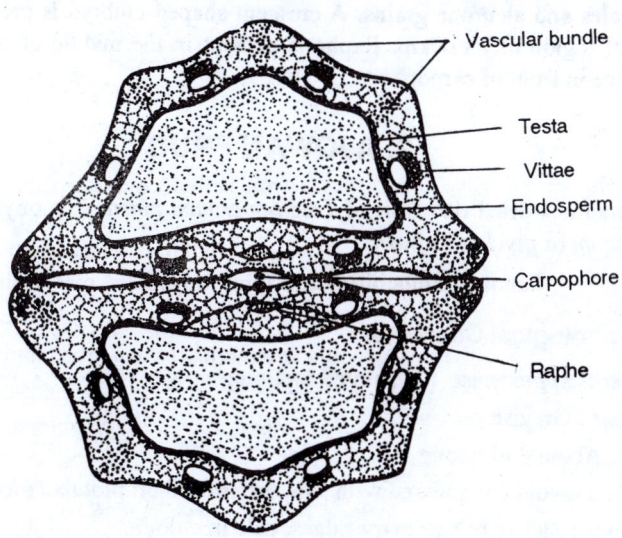

Fig. 7 (b) Fennel

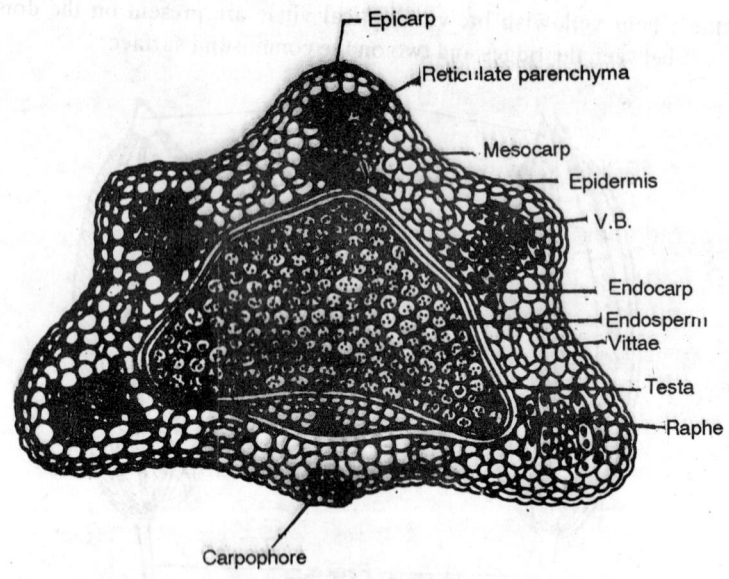

Fig. 7 (c) Fennel

Endocarp : It consist of narrow elongated cells with parquetry arrangement.

Testa : Single layered and yellowish colour.

Endosperm : It consist of polygonal parenchyma cells containing oil globules and aleurone grains. A crescent shaped embryo is present in the apical region of mericarp. Raphe is present in the middle of commisural surface in front of carpophore.

3. AJOWAN FRUIT

Ajowan is a dried ripe fruit of *Trachyspermum ammi* (Synonym : *Carum copticum* or *ptychotis ajwan*).

Family : Umbelliferae

Morphological Character

General Appearance : Separated mericrap

Colour : Greyish brown

Size : About 2 mm long

Shape : Ovoid compressed with pale coloured short protuberances

Surface : Shows five primary ridges, pale in colour

Odour : Thymol like

Taste : Characteristic aromatic

4. CARDAMOM

Cardamom is the dried ripe fruit of *Elettaria cardamomum* var minuscula and var major.

Family : Zingiberaceae

Morphological Characters

The fruit of cardamom is a capsule which is 1-2 cm long ovoid more or less three sided. The pericarp is dry and is 0.5 to 1 mm thick having woody texture. The capsule has three loculi with membramous septa and axile placentation. The seeds are about five to eight in number forming a single mass.

General Appearance : Inferior, trilocular capsule

Size : 1-2 cm long

Shape : Ovoid or oblong

Apex : Beaked·

Base : Round with remains of stalk

Surface : Smooth or longitudinally straited

Colour : Pale buff

Seeds : 5-8 in each capsule and attached in double rows with axile placentation in each of the three cell the capsule and are surrounded by arillus.

Size : Upto 4 mm in length, 3 mm in breadth

Shafic : Irregularly angular

Colour : Pale reddish brown

Surface : Transversely wrinkled. Number of tranverse wrinkles is useful in finding the different variety of cardamom. A longitudinal groove at one side indicate the position of raphe and in the depression at the end is the hilum. Different Varieties of the cardamom and their morphological characteristics:

1. *Aleppy Cardamom* : It is 8-10 mm long 4-10 mm wide having longitudinal striations. It is green in colour, pale buff when stored for long time.

2. *Mysore Cardamom* : It comes from Ceylon and is ovoid in shape having smooth surface and cream colour.

3. *Malabar Cordamon* : It also comes from Ceylon. The final is shorter more ovoid in shape having longitudinal wrinkles on the surface and hence it is less smooth than the Mysore variety.

4. *Mangalore Cardamom* : It is globular in shape.

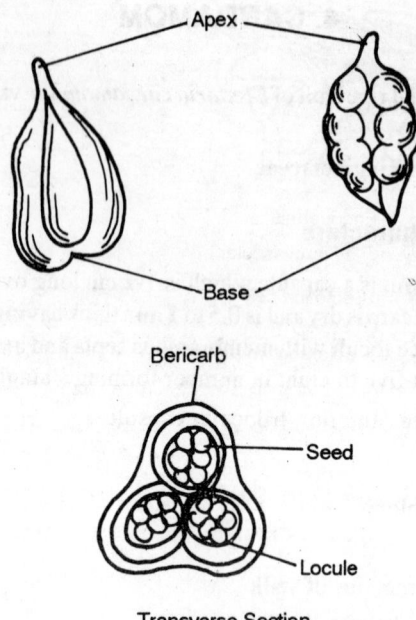

Transverse Section

Fig. 8. Cardamom

5. GINGER

Ginger consists of rhizome of *Zingiber officinale.*

Family : Zingiberaceae

Morphological Characters

General appearance : Sympodial branching of horizontal rhizome

Size : Length 5-15 cm., width 3-6 cm. and thickness 0.5 to 1.5 cm

Shape : Laterally flattened on the upper side with short flattened oblque obovate branches or fingers, each branch is 1 to 3 cm long and its apex show a depressed scar of the stem.

Surface : Longitudinally straited with occasional projecting fibres.

Fracture : Short, starchy, fibrous, fractured surface show a narrow bark, a well marked endodermis and a wide stele, showing numerous scattered greyish points (fibrovasculor bundles) and smaller yellowish point.

Colour : Buff

Odour : Agreeable and aromatic

Taste : Agreeable and pungent

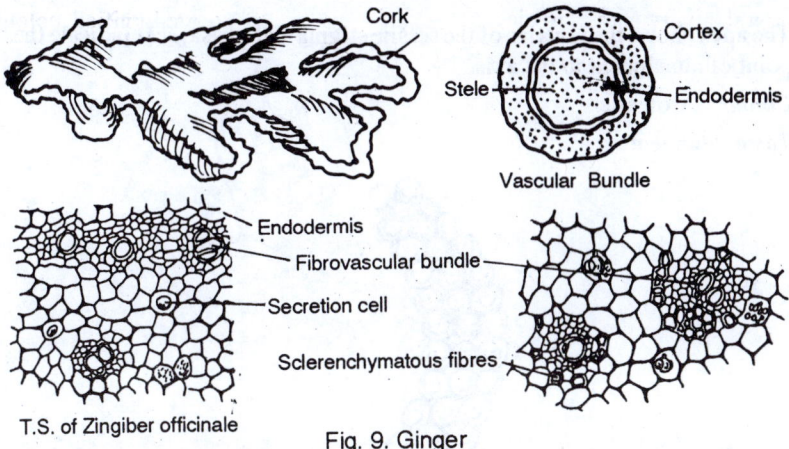

Fig. 9. Ginger

T.S. of Zingiber officinale

Microscopic Characters (Fig. 9a)

A T. S. of the rhizome shows the following tissue layer.

1. *Cork* : It consists of a outer zone of irregularly arranged cells and inner zone of radially arranged cells (about in Jamica Zinger).

2. *Cortex* : It consists of this walled, cellulosic round paranchyma cells with inter cellular spaces, containing starch grains, brown oleoresin cells are also present in the cortex.

3. *Vascular bundle* : Closed collateral fibro vascular bundles are also present in the cortex. In Stele ring of vascular bundles (without fibres) are present just below the endodermis. The xylem vessels have annular, spiral or reticulate thickening which are not lignified. The phloem fibres are thin walled with only central lumen lignified with pectosic transverse septa.

6. BLACK PEPPER

Black pepper consists of the dried unripe fruits of *Piper nigrum*.

Family : Piperaceae

Morphological Characters

General appearance : It is a entire round fruit

Shape : Almost globular

Size : 3.5-6 mm in diameter

Surface : The surface is dark brown or greyish black and strongly reticulated.

The apex shows the remains of the sessile stigma and a basal scar indicate the point of attachment to the axis.

Colour : Aromatic

Taste : Pungent

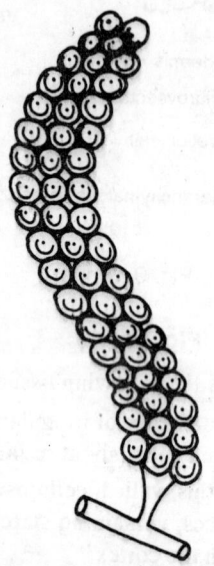

Fig. 10. Black pepper

7. ASAFOETIDA

Asafoetida is an oleo gum resin obtained from the rhizome and roots of *Ferula foetida, F. rubricaulis* and *F. asafoetida.*

Family : Umbelliferae

Morphological Character

Asafoetida occurs in three forms viz. paste, tear and bars (block or lump) Paste and tears are pure forms, but the bulk of the drug is mass.

1. **Tears :** These are separate, some more or less agglutinated together, are rounded or flattened and vary from 0.5 - 5 cm in diameter. They are of a dull yellow or sometime dingy-grey colour, some darken on keeping finally becoming reddish brown, but other retain their original colour for years. Probably the red variety is derived from *F. foetida,* the white from *F. rubricaulis.* When fresh they are usually tough at ordinary temparatures, becoming harder when cooled and soften when warmed. Internally they are yellowish or milky white, translucent or opaque.

The freshly exposed surface may pass through a very characteristic change of colour, becoming first pink, then red, and finally reddish brown, or may remain nearly white. The drug has an intense, pe trating, alliaceous odour and bitter, acrid, alliaceous taste.

2. **Mass :** Mass asafoetida consists of the tears agglutinated into a more or less uniform mass and mixed with varying quantities of extranceous substances such as stones, slices of the root, earthy matter, calcium carbonate, calcium sulphate etc., It is generally much inferior to the tears.

CHEMICAL TESTS

1. When triturated with water it forms yellowish-orange emulsion.
2. To the fractured surface, add sulphuric acid, a red or reddish brown colour is produced. When warmed with water the colour changes to violet.
3. Add to the fractured surface 50% nitric acid. Green colour is produced.
4. Combined umbelliferone test : Boil 0.5 g of drug and triturated with sand with 3 ml of concentrated hydrochloric acid and 3 ml of water for serveral minutes. Filter and to the filtrate add equal volume of alcohol and excess of strong solution of ammonia. A blue fluorescence is produced

    The test performed without hydrochloric acid will not show fluorescence.

I.P. standards :   1. Ash value not more than 15%
    2. Alcohol extractive value is less than 50%

8. NUTMEG

The drug is the kernel of dried ripe seeds of *Myristica fragrans* deprived of its arillus and seed coat.

    Family : Myristicaceac

Morphological Characters

The nutmeg fruits are ovoid about, 20 to 25 mm long and 1 to 28 mm wide. The kernel is greyish-brown externally and is marked with numerous minute dark reddish brown pointed lines, it is also reticulately marked with small furrows. This outer region is a thin layer of perisperm, which grows inwards into the endosperm at the position of the external furrows. The endosperm, which forms the bulk of the nutmeg, is greyish brown and is ruminated by the ingrowth of the dark brown perisperm. At one end of a nutmeg is small circular depression making the position of the radicle of the embryo; before the removal of the testa the hilum is immediately adjacent to the mark. A groove, marking the line of the raphe, extend, from the depression to the opposite end of the kernel where chalaza is situated. The embryo lies in a small cavity in the endosperm and its cotyledons gradually grow up in to endosperm as they absorb the food it contains. The cut surface of the nutmeg easily yields oil when indented with the finger nail.

Odour : Strong and aromatic

Taste : Aromatic and bitter.

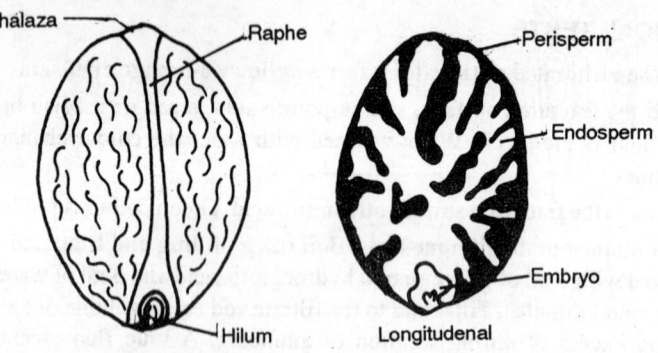

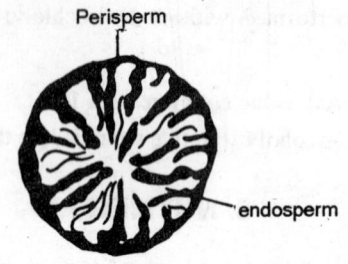

Fig. 11. Nutmeg

9. CINNAMON

The drug consists of the bark obtained from *Cinnamomum zeylanicum.*

Family : Lauraceae

Morphological Characters

General Appearance : It occurs as a single or compound quill

Size : About 1 meter, 6 - 10 mm in diameter, 0.5 mm thick

Outer Surface : It is yellowish brown showing longitudinal wavy lines, pericylic fibres and holes indicating the position of twigs.

Inner Surface : Dark brown in colour having longitudinal striation.

Fracture : Short and splintery

Odour : Aromatic

Taste : Warm, sweet aromatic.

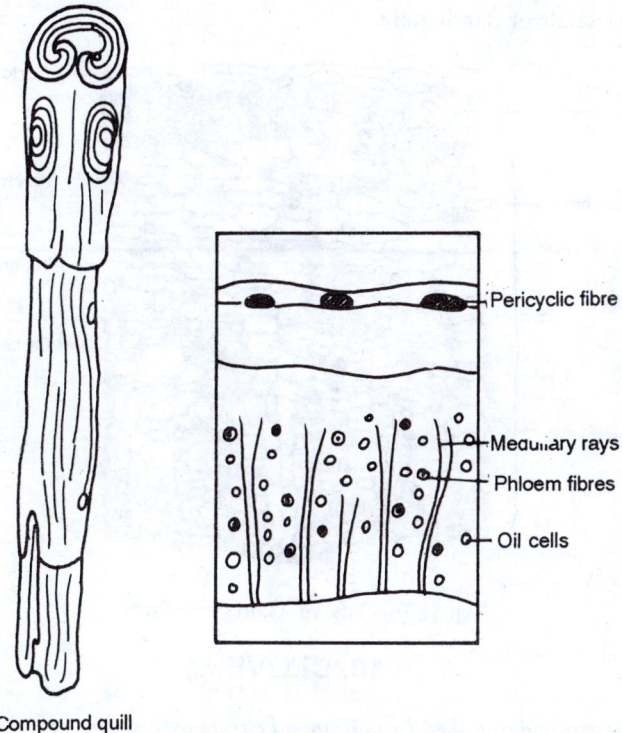

Compound quill

Fig. 12 (a) Cinnamon Bark

Microscopic Characters

At T.S. of the bark shows the following layers of tissues :

Cork : It consists of thin walled dark brown cell (if present, usually it is absent)

Sclereids : It is horse shoe shaped and are highly lignified.

Pericyclic Fibres : Lignified in group of 6 to 15.

Sieve Tubes : These are arranged in tangenitial bands which are completely collapsed in the outer layer.

Phloem Fibres : Occurs singly or in short tangenitial rows of two to five; they are lignified, colourless and slender.

Parenchyma : It consists of subrectangular cells which contain starch grain. Some cells also contain scattered minute needles of calcium oxalate.

Idioblast : There are longitudinally elongated cells containing volatile oil, or more rarely mucilage.

Medullay rays : There are usually biseriate, widening slightly as they approach to the pericycle. Many of these cell also contain minute needles of calcium oxalate or starch grain.

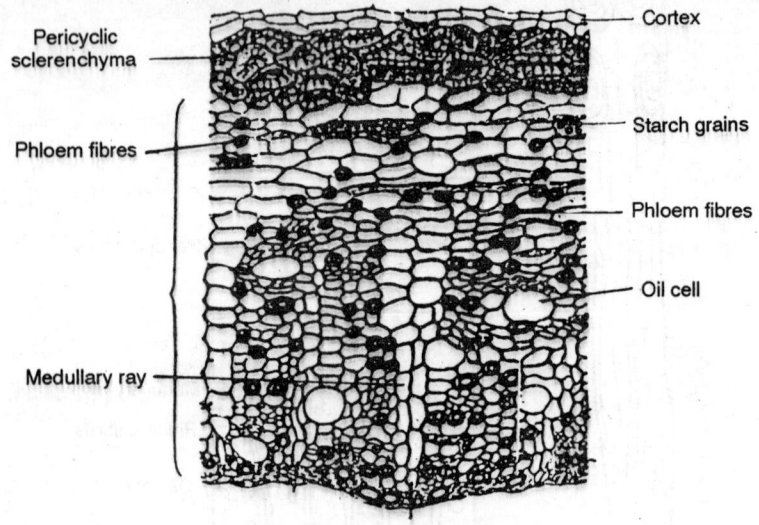

Fig. 12 (b) T.S. of Cinnamon Bark

10. CLOVE

It is a flower bud obtained from *Eugenia caryophyllus.*
              Family : Myrtaceae

Morphological Character

The flower bud is reddish brown in colour about 16-20 mm long and consists of lower solid stalk like portion called hypanthium and upper crown or cap.

Hypanthium : It is subcylindrical slightly flattened and tapering below. It is 10-13 cm long 4 cm wide and 2 mm thick.

Crown or Cap : It consists fo calyx, corolla, stamens and style. Calyx consists of four thick spreading projecting sepals. Corolla is dome shaped and is made up of four yellow coloured imbricate, immature, membranous petals and is called as head, crown or cap or dome.

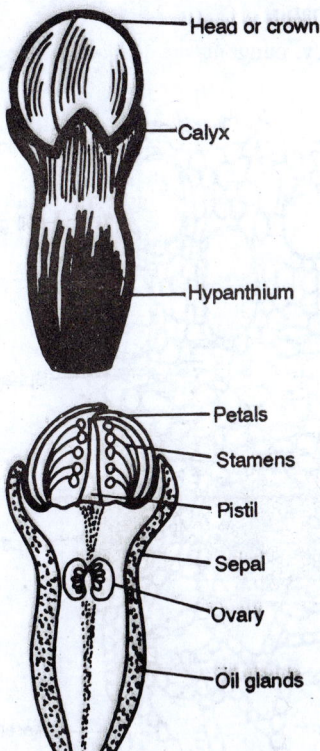

Fig. 13 (a) Clove

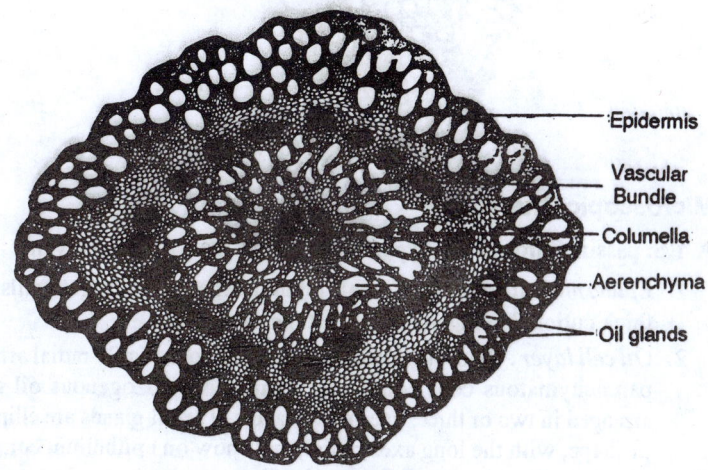

Fig. 13 (b) Clove

Odour : Pungent aromatic.

Taste : Aromatic, spicy, pungent

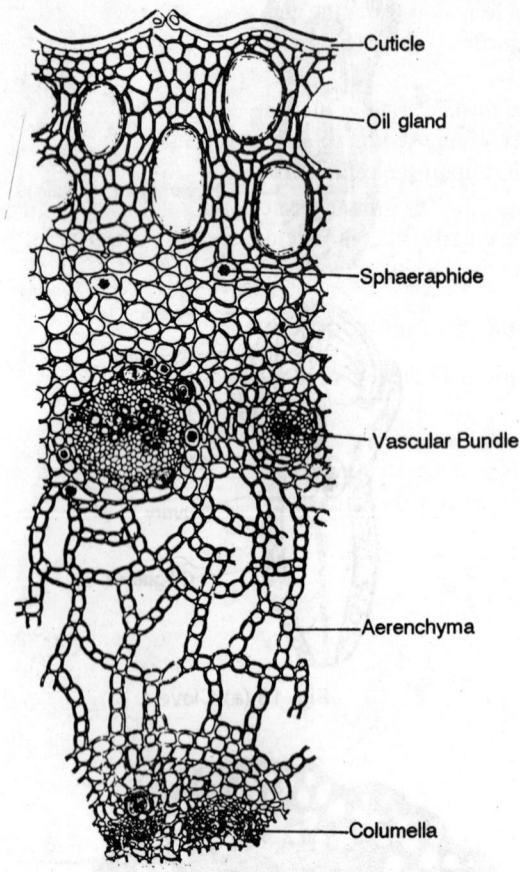

Fig. 13 (c) Clove

Microscopic Characters

A.T.S. passing through the hypanthium shows the following layers :

1. *Epidermis* : It consists of small tubular cells with straight walls and a thick cuticle having anomocytic type of stomata.

2. *Oil cell layer* : Below the epidermis is a zone of roughly radial arranged parenchymatous cells containing numerous schizogenous oil glands arranged in two or three, intermixed layers. The oil glands are ellipsoidal in shape, with the long axes radial, and show on epithelium composed of two or three layers of flattened cells.

The ground non parenchyma also contain clusture crystals of calcium oxalate.

3. *Vascular bundles* : A ring of bicollateral bundles is present in the paranchymatous layer the meristeles are enclosed in an incomplete ring of lignified fibre. The xylem is composed of 3-5 lignified spiral vessels.

4. *Aerenchyma* : Below the ring of vasular bundle is a zone of aerenchyma, composed of air spaces separated by lamellae one cell thick, which support the central columella.

5. *Columella* : The ground tissue of the columella is parenchymatous and is particularly rich in calcium oxalate crystals. In outer region of columella is a ring of some 17 small vascular bundles.

T.S. of hypanthium through ovary

The hypanthium, in the region of the ovary, show epidermis oil gland layer, ring of bicollateral bundles within this is a zone of cells with very slightly thickened cellulose walls limited internally by an inner epidermis forming the wall of the ovary. The dissepiment of ovary is parenchymatous, the placenta is are rich in calcium oxalate crystals and contain vascular bundles.

5

ASTRINGENTS

1. PALE CATECHU

Gambier, or pale catechu is dried aquous extract prepared from the leaves and young twigs of *Uncaria gambier.*

Family : Rubiaceae

Morphological Characters

Pale catechu occurs in cubes, each side of which is about 2.5 cm. Sometimes cubes are broken or attached to one another. The colour is reddish brown inner surface is porous and its colour is pale brown to buff. It has no odour and taste is astringent but some what bitter and latter sweet.

When mounted in water catechu shows minute acicular crystals of catechin, many of which are branched and interlacing. They dissolve on warming and leave considerable amount of debris.

CHEMICAL TESTS

1. **Gambier fluorescin test :** Boil a little powdered drug with alcohol, filter and add sodium hydroxide solution to the filterate, stir and add few ml of light petroleum. Petroleum layer shows green fluorescence. (Black catechu does not show this test)

2. Heat about 0.5 gm of powdered drug with 5 ml of chloroform in a dish and evaporate the filtrate on water bath. A greenish yellow residue is left due to the presence of chlorophyll in the drug. In black catechu this test is negative because there is no chlorophyll present in it.

3. **Match stick test :** Dip the wooden match stick in the solution of the drug and dry it over a flame. Moisten the stick with hydrochloric acid

and warm, purple colour appear on the match stick due to the conversion of catechin into phloroglucinol. (this test is also positive in black catechu).

4. **Vanillin hydrochloric acid test :** Make solution containing vanillin 1 ml, alcohol 10 ml and dilute hydrochloric acid 10 ml. This test also gives pink or red colour due to the formation of phloroglucinol. This test is also positive in black catechu.

2. BLACK CATECHU

It is the dried aqueous extract prepared from the heart wood of *Acacia catechu*.

Family : Leguminosae

Morphological Characters

Black catechu occurs in irregular black or brownish black mass. Outer surface firm and brittle and shows covering of leaves. When broken, the fractured surface appears glassy and porous and sometime it is soft. It has no odour and taste is bitter.

CHEMICAL TEST

Match stick and vanillin hydrochloric acid test are positive while Gambier fluorescin test is negative in black catechu.

DRUGS ACTING ON NERVOUS SYSTEM

1. HYOSCYMUS

Hyoscymus is the dried leaves and flowering tops of *Hyoscymus niger* containing not less than 0.05 percent of the alkaloids of hyoscymus calculated as hyoscyamine.

Family : Solanaceae

Morphological Characters

Leaves

Size : Annual leave, about 10 cm long 1st year biennial 20-30 cm long 2nd year biennial 5-25 cm long.

Shape : Oblong ovate or triangular ovate, First year leaves are ovate lanceolate.

Margin : Irregularly toothed, sinuate and in some cases, particularly 2nd year biennial, pinnatified, Annual leaves are often less prominently toothed.

Apex : Acute

Base : Mostly sessile, annual and first year biennial leaves with a petiole, in the latter upto 30 cm long.

Veins : Broad, pale conspicuous midrib, and several prominent viens, all covered with long hairs, these are less dense on annual leaves.

Flower

The flower occur solitary or in small cymes. In the biennial plant the lower flowers are shortly stalked in the forks of the branches, and the upper ones in one sided leafy spikes rolled back when in bud, in axils of large, hairy bracts.

(a) *Calyx* : Gamosepalous, five lobed, hairy, persistent, increases in size when the fruit forms.

(b) *Corolla* : Gamopetalous, about 2.5 cm long pale, dingy yellow with purple veins, shortly funnel shaped five lobed   (Annual henbane exhibits fewer, pale purple veins), 5 epipetalous stamens.

(c) Fruit : The ovary is superior, two celled with numerous ovules, the stigma is capitate and two lobed. An almost globular pysidium surrounded by the calyx, which develops after fertilization until about 2.5 cm long, with 5 stiff pointed lobes protruding above the fruit, contain numerous seeds about 1 mm in length and breadth which are reniform in shape with a light brown reticulate seed coat.

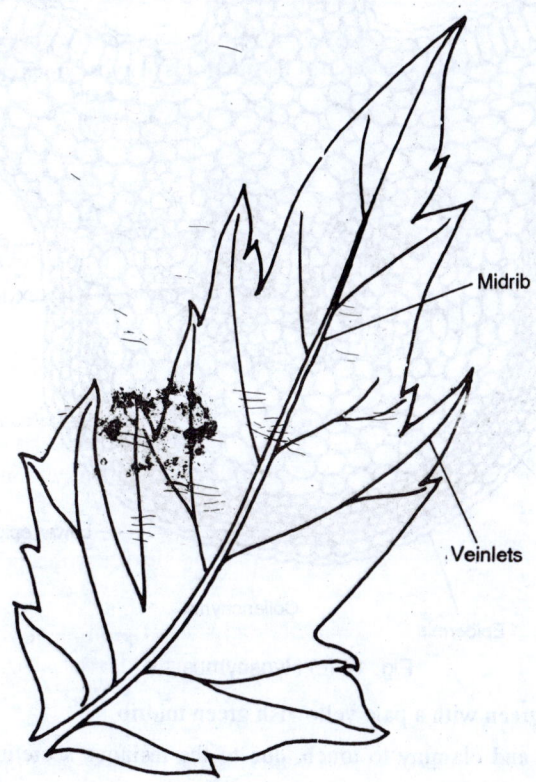

Fig. 14 (a) Hyoscymus

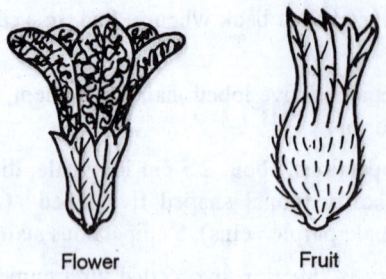

Flower   Fruit

Fig. 14 (b) Hyoscymus

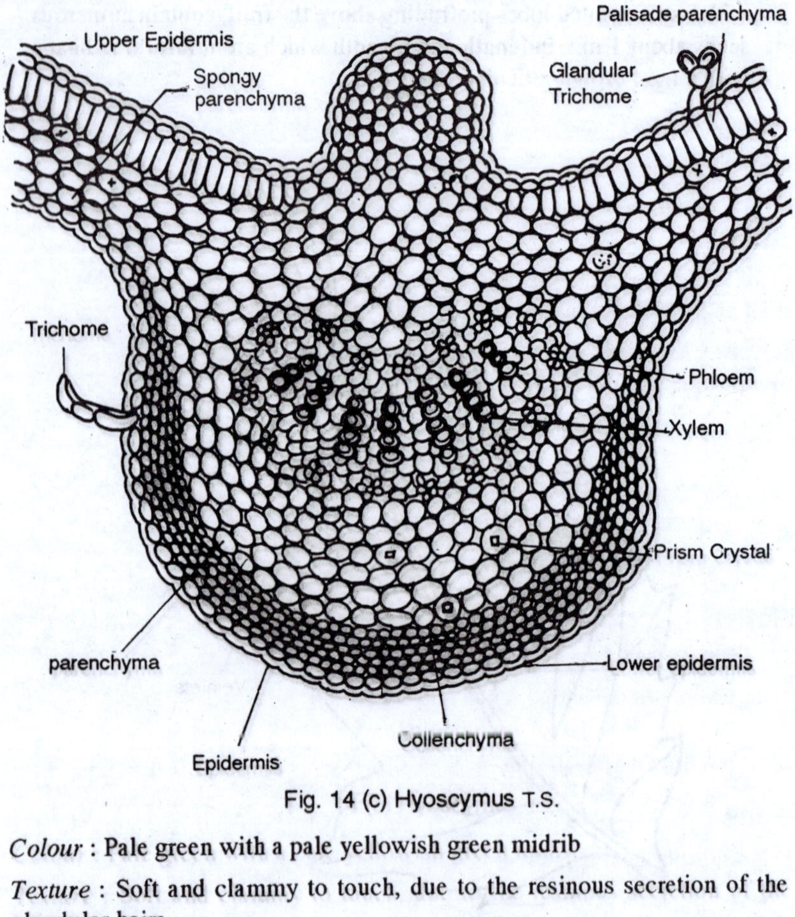

Palisade parenchyma

Upper Epidermis

Spongy parenchyma

Glandular Trichome

Trichome

Phloem

Xylem

Prism Crystal

parenchyma

Lower epidermis

Epidermis

Collenchyma

Fig. 14 (c) Hyoscymus T.S.

Colour : Pale green with a pale yellowish green midrib

Texture : Soft and clammy to touch, due to the resinous secretion of the glandular hairs.

Taste : Bitter

Odour : Strong and characteristic, especially noticeable when the drug is fresh or has been stored in the closed container.

2. BELLADONNA

The drug consist of the leaves and other aerial parts of *Atropa belladonna Linn.* Indian belladonna is obtained from *Atropa acuminata.*

Family : Solanaceae

Morphological character

Leaf

Size : The larger leaf from 8-20 cm. The smaller upto 5 cm

Shape : Broadly ovate

Margin : Entire

Apex : Acuminate

Base : Tapering, stout, straight petiole upto 4 cm long, lamina is somewhat decurrent

Veins : Midrib and lateral veins very distinct. Lateral veins leave the midrib at an angle of about 60° and curve towards the apex.

Surface : Glabrous shows numerous prominence of idioblast of calcium oxalate crystal.

STEM

1. Green to purplish green
2. Slightly flattened with one or two deep grooves
3. Leaves are alternate

Flowers

1. Small drooping, about 2-5 cm long and pedicillate.
2. Calyx : Persistent, 5 lobed and companulate.
3. Corolla : Five lobed, companulate when fresh, dull purplish in colour, but brown after drying.

Fruits

1. Subspherical berries, 3-10 mm in diameter
2. Derived from bilocular ovary containing numerous ovules with axile placentation
3. Seeds small, sub-reniform with brown reticulation.

The plant is perennial herb about 1.5 meter in height. Root is fleshy tapering and bears numerous rootlets. Stem is straight, herbaceous, branched, glabrous or slightly hairy, leaves are alternate.

Odour : Slight

Taste : Bitter and unpleasant

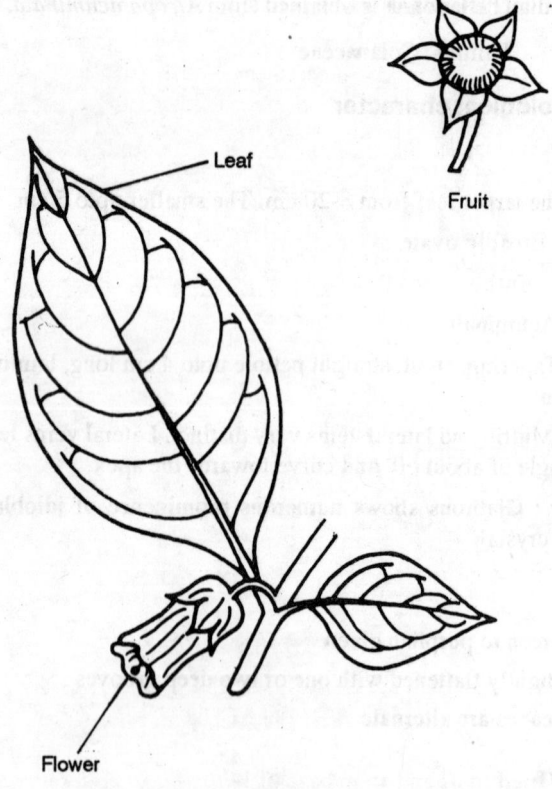

Fig. 15 Belladonna

3. ACONITE

It is the dried roots of *Aconitum napellus* Linn.

Family : Ranunculaceae

Morphological Characters

Size, form and Surface characters : 4-10 cm long, 1-3.5 cm at crown, from which it narrows sharply, conical and with longitudinal wrinkles' usually slightly twisted Numeorus scars where rootlets have broken off are present.

Fracture : Short

Fractured surface : Starchy

Odour : None

Taste : Bitter, afterwards gives peristent tingling sensation

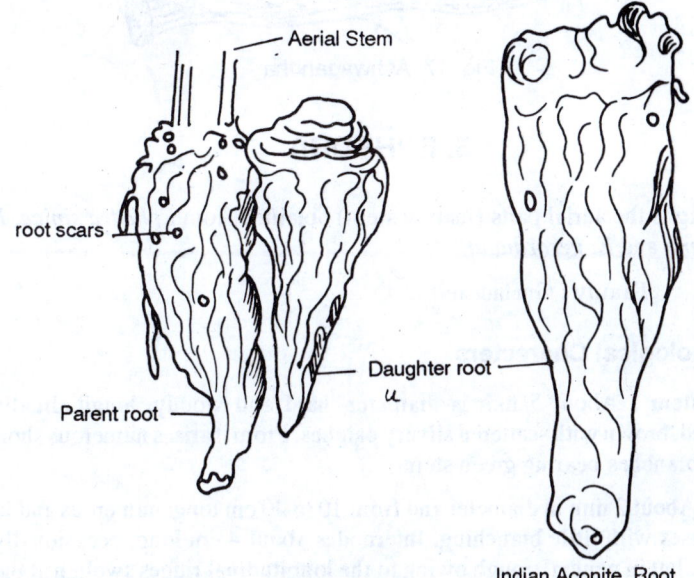

Fig. 16. Aconite

4. ASHWAGANDHA

It is the dried roots and stem base of *Withania somnifera*.

Family : Solanaceae

Morphological Characters

The young roots are straight, unbranched and conical and are available in the market in different length. Thickness varies according to age usually below 5-12 mm

Colour : Outer surface is buff to greyish yellow having longitudinal wrinkles.

Fracture : Short

Fractured surface : Creamish

Odour : Characteristic

Taste : Slightly bitter

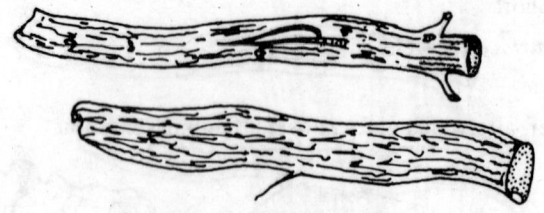

Fig. 17. Ashwagandha

5. EPHEDRA

The durg is the aerial parts (mainly stem) obtained from *Ephedra sinica, E equisetina* and *E. gerardiana.*

Family : Gnetaceae

Morphological Characters

Main stem : About 5 mm is diameter, hard and woody, longitudinally wrinkled, brown with scattered silvery patches. From it arises numerous short brown branches bearing green stem.

Stem : About 2 mm in diameter and from 10 to 40 cm long; numerous and in most cases with little branching, Internodes about 4 cm long; occasionally smooth, but in general rough owing to the longitudinal ridges swollen at the nodes Colour is green, but on long storing may turn yellow. Drug collected in winter is grey.

Leaves : Greatly reduced, the lamina is 2-4 mm long, in pairs at the nodes, fused at the base and thus encircling the stem as a sheath 2-3 mm deep, apex is acute and recurved. The apex is white and the base is brown, but paler in the upper part of the stem.

6. OPIUM

Opium is the latex obtained by making incision on the unripe capsules of *Papaver somniferum* Linn., dried or partly dried by heat or spontaneous evaporation and worked out into some what irregularly shaped massess or moulded into masses of uniform size and shape.

Family : Papaveraceae

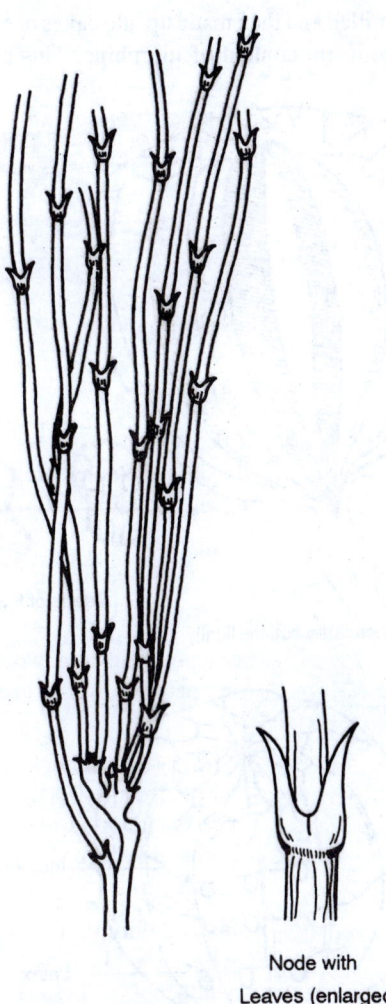

Node with
Leaves (enlarged)

Fig. 18. Ephedra

Morphological Characters

The cakes of opium formed by the collection in the field have shapes which
are rounded, conical, irregular or flattened and vary much in weight from
about 50 g to serveral kilograms and they may or may not be covered with
poppy leaves. This form of opium is usually referred to as "natural" opium
and does not come into regular commerce. The government of the countries
in which opium is prepared have established monopolies in the opium trade
and cakes for export are prepared in controlled factories where the "natural"

opium is mixed and milled and then made up into cakes of some definite shape containing a fairly uniform content of morphine. This opium is known as manipulated opium.

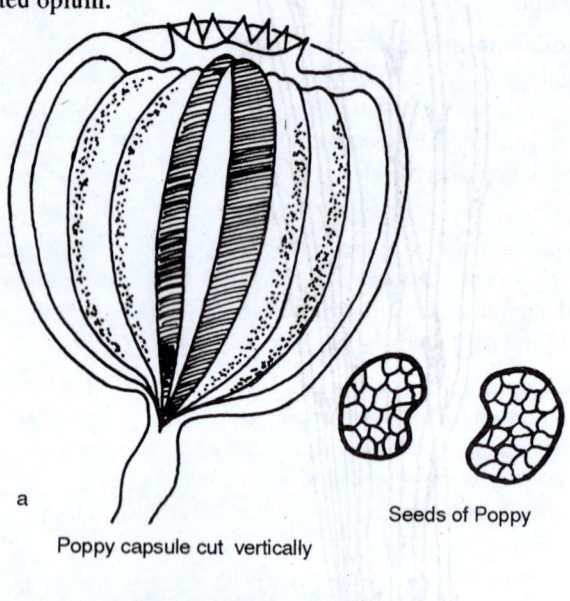

a

Poppy capsule cut vertically

Seeds of Poppy

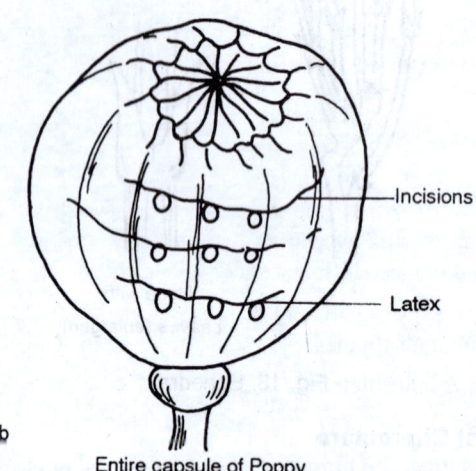

b

Entire capsule of Poppy

Incisions

Latex

Fig. 19. (a) & (b))Opium

(i) **Turkish opium :** It occurs in subcylindrical cakes about 9 cm high and 15 cm in diameter, coated with coarsely powdered poppy leaves, giving them a greenish grey mottled appearance, a circular official label is attached to the side of each cake. The opium has a uniform slightly granular texture and a pale chocolate brown colour; it is moderately plastic when fresh but becomes firm and even hard when kept for sometime.

(ii) **Yugoslavian opium :** It occurs as oblong cakes with rounded ends each weighing 160 to 225 g the cakes are about 18 to 20 cm by 6 to 7.5 cm by 1.5 to 2.4 cm. Externally they are either coated with broken poppy leaf and are greyish green in colour or they are devoid of poppy leaf and are dark brown. The interior is uniform in texture and dark brown in colour.

(iii) **Persian or Iranian opium :** It occurs in brick-shaped cakes about 10 by 5 by 7 cm each wraped in red paper. At times the opium has been moulded into other forms such as conical masses and short sticks. It is brittle and dark reddish brown in colour.

(iv) **Indian opium :** It occurs in block which are very dark brown or nearly black and internally are smooth and homogeneous. It also occurs in cubical blocks about 8 to 9 cm edge, each weighing about 2 lb and wrapped in two sheets of thin white paper and tied with string. More recently block are packed in polythene bags.

7. CANNABIS

Cannabis consists of dried flowering tops of pistillate plants of *Cannabis sativa* Linn.

Family : Moraceae

Description

Stem : It is straight with ascending branches, all longitudiarlly furrowed bearing fruits and cymose inflorescence.

Bracts : Simple sessile or palmately compound with three leaflets and each has two small subulate stiputes.

Shape : Lamina is lanceolate.

Margin : Entire

Size : 15-20 mm long, 2-4 mm wide

Lower bracts are larger, palmately compound with 3-5 leaflets.

Shape : Lanceolate

Margin : Serrate

Bracteoles : Two boat shaped bracteoles enclosing single pistillate flower are seen.

Flower : It consists of ovary enclosed by perianth. It is about 2 mm long. Two reddish brown stigma can be seen with a lens.

Fruits : Few fruits are present which are 5-6 mm long 4 mm wide and ovoid in shape.

Odour : Powerful.

Taste : Almost tasteless.

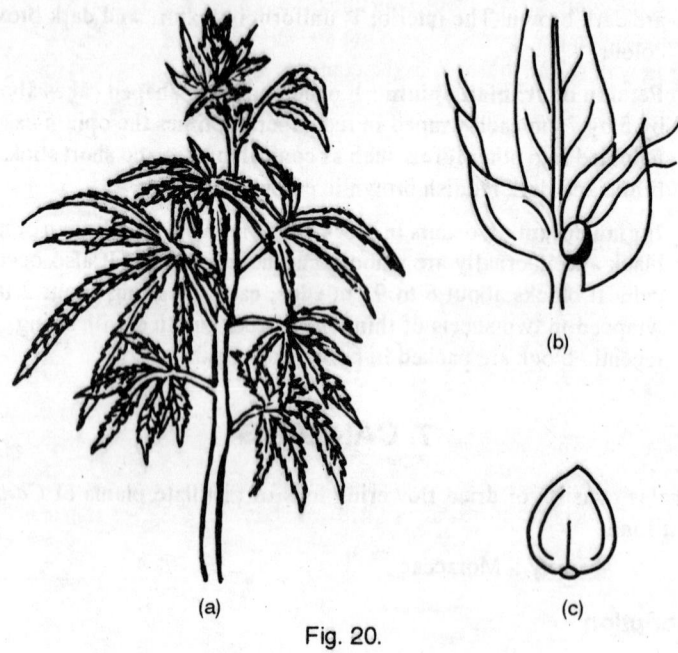

(a)

(b)

(c)

Fig. 20.

(a) Cannabis herb
(b) Bract and bracteole opened to show flower
(c) Fruit of cannabis

8. NUX VOMICA

The drug consists of the seeds of *Strychnos nux-vomica* Linn.

Family : Loganiaceae

Morphological Characters

General appearance : The seeds are disc shaped and thick. They are usually not quite flat but are little depressed on one side and arched on the other side, or some time irregularly bent.

Size : 20-25 mm in diameter and 4 mm thick

Colour : Ash grey or greenish grey

Outer surface : The outer surface is covered with numerous, closely appressed trichomes which radiate from centre to the circumference. The edge of seed is somewhat rounded. At one point on the margin where the micropyle is situated, there is distinct prominence from which a raised line passes to the centre of the seed. This line does not exists in the fresh seed, but makes it appearance during the drying and disappears when the dry seed is soaked in water. The hilum is in the centre of either the raised or depressed surface.

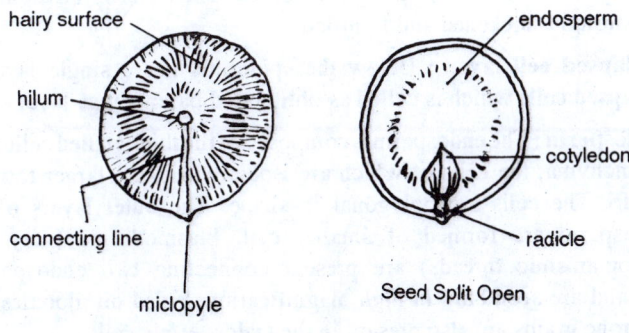

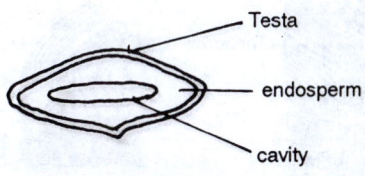

T.S. cut to flat Surface

Fig. 21 (a) Nuxvomica

L.S. OF THE SEED

The L.S. of the seed shows horny endosperm about 2 mm thick. A central narrow disc shaped cavity which is about 16 to 20 mm in diameter and upto 1.5 mm wide is also seen. The endosperm is perforated above the micropyle by a cylindrical channel leading to the disc shaped hollow and enclosing the terete radicle of the embryo. Attached to the radicle and lying within the hollow are two cordate leafy cotyledons having a distinct palmate venation with five to seven veins. The cotyledons are about 5 to 6 mm long and the radicle about 4 mm. The endosperm is translucent grey in colour and the embryo is whitish.

Odour : None

Taste : Persistent and intense bitter taste.

T.S. OF NUX VOMICA SEED

The T.S. of the seed show the following layers :

1. **Epidermis :** The epidermal cells are extended to form appressed trichomes which are 600 to 1000 μ long and about 25 μ in diameter. The basal position is about 75 μ high and broad. The walls of the trichomes are strongly thickened and lignified.

2. **Collapsed cell layer :** Below the epidermis lies a single layer of collapsed cells which is called as obliterated parenchyma layer.

3. **Endosperm :** The endosperm is composed of the thick walled cellulosic parenchyma, the cells of which are isodiametric, are larger towards inside. The cells are polygonal in shape. The outer layers of the endosperm are formed of smaller cell. Plasmodesma (very fine protoplamsmic threads) are present connecting two endospermic cell and are seen only in high magnification. Fixed oil globules and aluerone grains are also present in the endospermic cells.

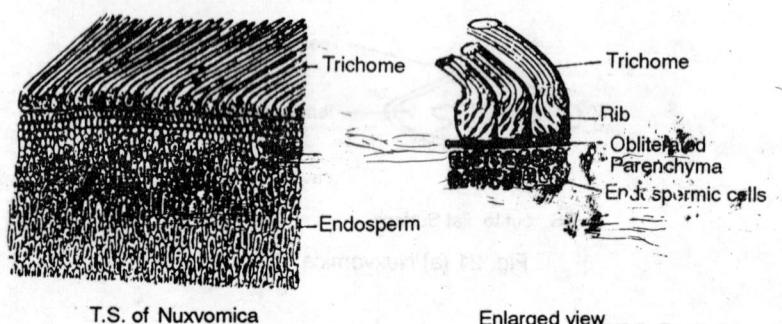

T.S. of Nuxvomica   Enlarged view

Fig. 21 (b) Nuxvomica

Chemical Test for Strychnine

Cut a thick T.S. of the seed and to it add few drops of sulphovanadic acid (1% solution of ammonium vendate in concentrated sulphuric acid) a purple colour appears due to the presence of strychnine.

Chemical Test for Brucine

To another thick T.S. of the seed add a drop of concentrated nitric acid, an orange red colour shows the presence of brucine in the seed.

7

ANTIHYPERTENSIVES

1. RAUWOLFIA

Rauwolfia consists of the dried root and rhizome of *Rauwolfia serpentina* Benth.

Family : Apocynaceae

Morphology of Root and Rhizome

In external characters pieces of rhizome and of root closely resemble one or another and the only reliable method of distinction is to find out the small central pith of the rhizome having a diameter of only 1 to 2 mm as seen in the smoothed transversely cut surface.

Shape : The roots and rhizome are sub cylindrical or slightly tapering, somewhat tortuous and rarely branched, pieces of the rhizomes are less uniform in diameter.

Size : The majority of the pieces of the drugs are about 8 to 15 cm long and 0.5 to 1 cm thick some pieces are as much as 40 cm long and may be upto 2 cm thick. Some pieces are as much as 40 cm long and may be upto 2 cm in diameter.

Colour : The outer surface is dull and greyish brown

Outer Surface : The outer surface shows faint longitudinal ridges. In older pieces it is somewhat scaly and the bark exfoliate in small patches, short length of aerial stem are attached to some pieces of the drug.

Fracture : Short and the fractured surface show a pale yellowish white, finely radiate and compact wood, which occupies about three quarters of the diameter and has 3 to 8 growth rings.

Odour : Odour less

Taste : Bitter taste

Fluorescence test : A one percent tincture of the drug gives blue fluorescence in u.v. light.

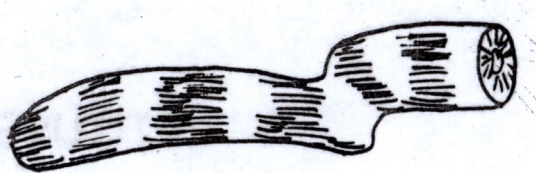

Fig. 22. Rauwolfia

8

ANTITUSSIVES

1. VASAKA

The drug consists of the leaves of *Adhatoda vasica* Nees.

Family : Acanthaceae

Morphological Characters of Leaves

Size : 10-20 cm long and 3.5 to 6 cm broad

Shape : Entire, lanceolate, markedly acute at the base and slightly acuminate towards the apex.

Petiole : Short about 2 cm long

Venation : Pinnate

Colour : Dull brownish green

Odour : Slightly characteristic

Taste : Somewhat bitter

2. BALSAM OF TOLU

Balsam of Tolu is balsam obtained by making incision in the trunk of *Myroxylon balsamum* Linn.

Family : Leguminosae

Description of Balsam of Tolu

General Appearance : The fresh balsam of Tolu in a soft tenacious, resinous mass which takes the form of the vessel in which it is kept. By keeping it gradually hardens.

Colour : It is yellowish brown when fresh and brown when it is kept for longer period.

Other characters : It can be easily powdered, it softens when warmed.

Odour : It has agreeable fragrant balsamic odour.

Taste : It has balsamic taste and adheres to the teeth when chewed.

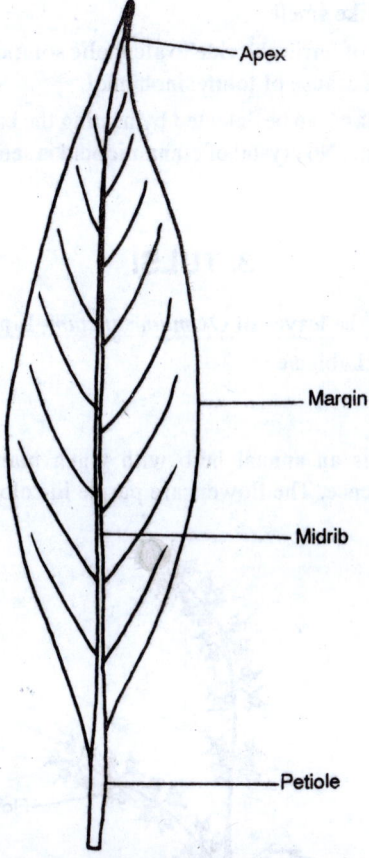

Fig.23. Vasaka Leaf

A small piece warmed and pressed into a thin film between two glass slides exhibits, when examined by microscope, colourless crystals of cinnamic acid embedded in a transparent mass.

Solubility : It is easily soluble in alcohol, acetone and chloroform but partially soluble in carbon disulphide.

CHEMICAL TESTS

1. Dissolve 1 g of tolu balsam in 10 ml of alcohol by heating. The solution

shows acidic reaction with litmus and insoluble residue is not more than 4%.

2. Boil 1 g of balsam with 5 ml water and filter. To the filtrate add 3 ml of 1% aqueous potassium permanganate solution and heat. Cinnamic acid present in the balsam is oxidized to benzaldehyde showing the bitter almond like smell.

3. Add few drops of ferric chloride to alcoholic solution of balsam. Green colour is seen because of toluresinotannol.

4. Exhausted balsam can be detected by heating the balsam and making a thin film on slide. No crystal of cinnamic acid is seen on the slide under microscope.

3. TULSI

The drug consists of the leaves of *Ocimum sanctum* Linn.

Family : Labiatae

CHARACTERS

The plant of Tulsi is an annual herb with much branched stem having verticillate inflorescence. The flowers are purple in colour in recemes.

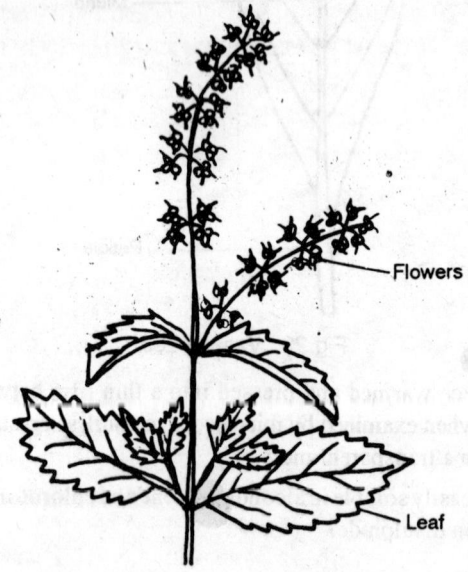

Fig. 24. Tulsi plant

Leaves

Shape : The leaves are petiolate and are oblong, exstipulate

Apex : Acute

Margin : entire or serrate

Trichomes : Present on both surface and are minutely glandular dotts are seen

Odour : Aromatic

Taste : Pungent

ANTIRHEUMATICS

1. GUGGAL

Guggal is the oleogum resin obtained from the bark of *Commiphora mukul.*
Hook-ex-stock

Family : Burseraceae

Morphology of Various Parts of Plant

Stem and bark

Young stem : Glandular pubescent brownish.

Old stem : Brownish to pale yellow covered with papery layers of dead cork cells.

Bark : Greenish colour, thick containing schizolysigenous oil glands embedded in the phloem region.

Leaves : 1-4 foliate, subsessile leaflets

Shape : Ovate

Margin : Serrate

Surface : Smooth and shining

Flowers : They are present in fasicles of 2-3 with short pedicle

Calyx : Campanulate, traingular, 4-5 in number, glandular and hairy

Petals : brownish red, linear

Stamens : 8-10

Style : Single

Fruits : Drupe, red, ovoid, acute, and readily splitting.

Oleogumresin : It is available in the form of irregular pieces weighing about 250 g.

Surface : Greenish brown or reddish yellow and powdery

Fracture : Splintery and translucent occasionally with whitish marks

Odour : Aromatic

Taste : Bitter and acrid

Total ash : 7.90 - 8.20

Acid value : 4.50 - 4.81

Specific gravity : 0.83 - 0.87

2. COLCHICUM

The drug consists of seeds and corms of *Colchicum autumnale* Linn.

Indian drug is obtained from *Colchicum luteum* Baker.

Family : Liliaceae

Morphology of the seed

Shape : Colchicum seeds are sub-spherical

Size : About 2-3 mm in diameter.

Outer surface : The testa is dull and dark reddish brown, minutely pitted and rough. Over the raphe, which extends for a quarter of the circumference of the amphitropous seed, there is a local enlargement, the strophiole, at the end of which is a pointed projection at the hilum.

Odour : None

Taste : Unpleasantly bitter.

Morphology of Corm

Shape : The fresh corm is bluntly conical and flattened on one side. The dried slices are sub-reniform to oval in shape.

Size : The fresh corm is 3.5 to 4 cm high, 2.5 to 3 cm wide and about 2 cm thick. The dried slices are from 2 to 5 mm thick and about 3 cm wide.

Outer surface : Near the base of the flat surface is a shallow depression containing a bud in the fresh corm. At one end of the corm is the scar of the stem. The scars of the fibrous root are present at the base. Internally it is firm, white and fleshy.

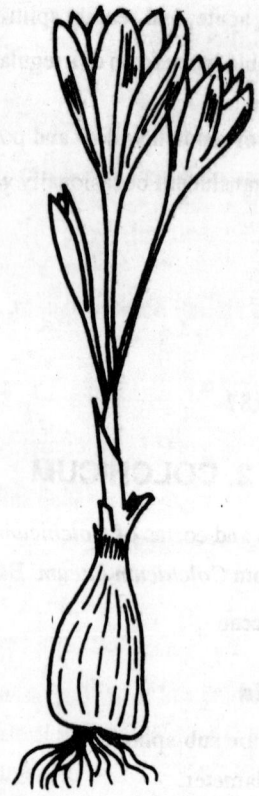

Colchicum corm with flower

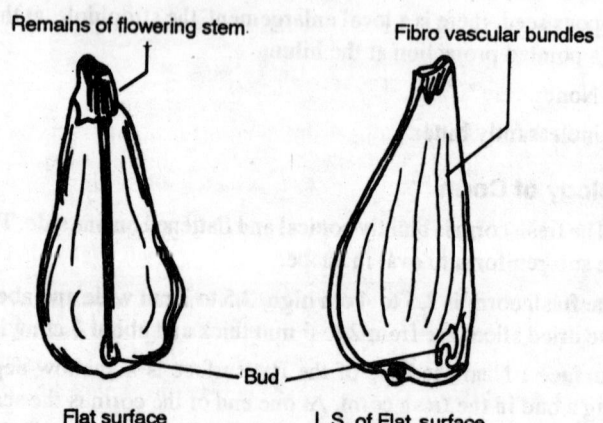

Remains of flowering stem.

Fibro vascular bundles

Bud

Flat surface

L.S. of Flat surface

Fig. 25. Colchicum

The surface of the dried slices shows the groove on one side being due to the shrinkage of the more aqueous parenchyma occuring in the centre of the straight edge. The surface of the edge of the slice is dark brown, the transverse surface shows a white, mealy ground tissue.

Odour : The fresh corm has disagreeable odour. While the dried corm is odourless.

Taste : It has bitter taste.

ANTITUMOUR

VINCA

Vinca is the dried whole plant of *Catharanthus roseus* G. Don.

Family : Apocynaceae

Morphological Characters

It is a herbacious shrub. The plant is about one meter high and has woody texture at base.

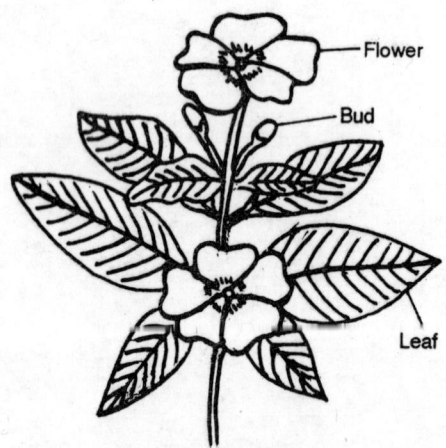

Fig. 26. Vinca plant

Leaves : Simple, arranged oppositely.

Shape : Oblong with a petiolate acute base.

Apex : Rounded or mucronate.

Margin : Entire

Flowers : Solitary, pink, white or violet in colour.

11

ANTILEPROTIC

CHAULMOOGRA OIL

Chaulmoogra oil is the fixed oil obtained by cold expression from the fresh, ripe seeds of *Hydnocarpus kurzii* (King) Warb.

Family : Flacourtiaceae

CHARACTERS

The oil is yellow or brownish yellow liquid. Below 25°, it is whitish soft solid.

Odour : Characteristic resembling that of rancid butter.

Taste : Somewhat acrid

Solubility : It is sparingly soluble in alcohol; soluble in chloroform and in solvent ether.

Weight per ml : 0.935 to 0.960 g. (at 25°C)

Specific rotation : Specific rotation is determined by dissolving 10 g in chloroform and diluting to 100 ml with the same solvent, not less than +48° and not more than +60°.

Acid value : Not more than 13

Iodine value : 93 to 104

Saponification value : 196 to 213.

12

ANTIDIABETICS

PTEROCARPUS

It is the juice obtained from incisions in the trunk of *Pterocarpus marsupium* Roxburgh. It is also called Malabar kino. African kino is offained from *Pterocarpus erinaceous.* Poiret,

Family : Leguminosae

CHARACTERS

Occurs in small, glistening, angular grains

Size : 3-5 mm in diameter

Colour : Black, edges appear transparent and dark red

Fracture : Hard brittle breaking with vitreous fracture.

Odour : None

Taste : Astringent when chewed, adheres to the teeth, colouring the saliva red.

Solubity in water : 80-90%.

2. GYMNEMA SYLVESTRE

It is also called Gurmar or Madhunashini in Hindi.

It is the herb of *Gymnema sylvestre.*

Family : Asclepidiaceae.

General morphology of the plant

It is a woody climber.

Leaves are opposite usually ovate or elliptic in shape.

Length : Varies from 1.25-2.0 inch and breadth 0.5-1.25 inch. It bears small yellow flowers in umbellate cyme. Follictel tesete lanceolate, upto 3 inch length.

13

DIURETICS

1. GOKHRU

There are two type of Gokhru available from two different plants. The small Gokhru is the fruit obtained from *Tribulus terrestris* Linn.

Family : Zygophyllaceae

The large Gokhru is the fruit obtained from *Pedalium murex.*

Family : Pedaliaceae

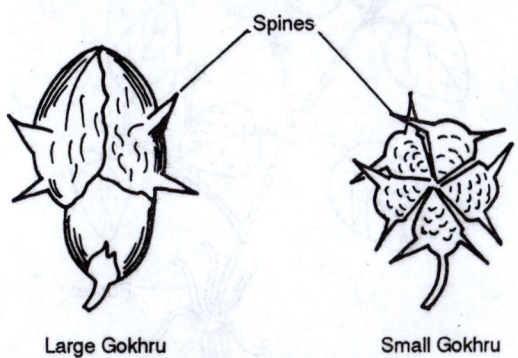

Fig. 27. Small & Large Gokhru

CHARACTERS OF SMALL GOKHRU

Shape : Globose

Colour : Yellowish white

Outer surface : The outer surface of the fruit is spiny having five woody, spiny cocci and each coccus has four pointed rigid spines. Two of the larger spines are directed towards the apex and the other two smaller ones are directed downwards. Each coccus contains several seeds.

CHARACTERS OF LARGE GOKHRU

Shape : It has pyramid ovoid shape tapering at the base and apex.

Colour : Brown

Outer surface : Each fruit has four spines and does not show separate cocci.

2. PUNARNAVA

Punarnava consists of the fresh or the dried plant, *Boerhaavia diffusa* Linn.

Family : Nyctaginaceae

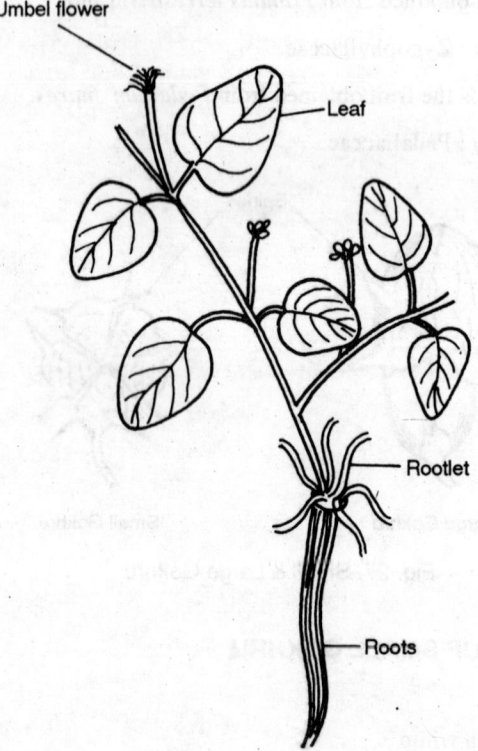

Fig. 28. Punarnava

CHARACTERS

Stem : Greenish purple, stiff, slender, cylindrical, thickened at nodes, minutely pubescent or nearly glabrous, prostrate or ascending, divaricately branched, branches from common stalk, often more than a yard long.

Leaves : Opposite in unequal pairs, larger ones 25 to 37 mm long and smaller ones 12 to 18 mm long, ovate-oblong or suborbicular, apex rounded or slightly pointed, base subcordate or rounded green and glabrous above, whitish below, margin entire or undulate, turned up and pinkish in certain cases, rather thick in texture; petioles; nearly as long as the blade, slender.

Flowers : Very small in size, nearly sessile or shortly stalked 10 to 25 cm in small umbels arranged on slender long stalks; bracteoles; small, acute perianth, tube constricted above the ovary; lower part greenish, ovoid, ribbed, upper part pink, funnel shapped, 3 mm long, tube 5 lobed; stamens 2 to 3.

Fruit : One seeded nut, 6 mm long, clavate, 5 ribbed, viscidly glandular.

14

ANTIDYSENTERICS

1. IPECACUANHA

Ipecacuanha consists of the dried, enlarged adventitious roots of *Cephaelis ipecacuanha* (Brot.) A Rich.

Family : Rubiaceae

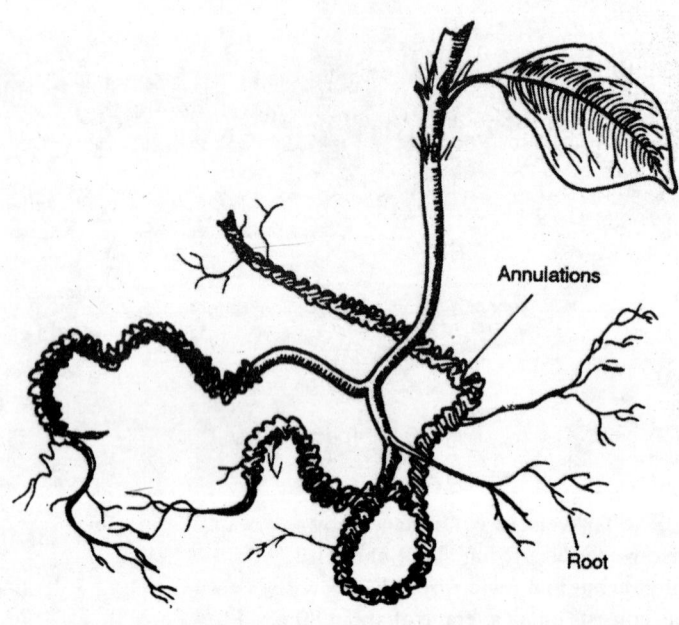

Fig. 29 (a) Ipecacuanha Root

Morphological Characters

Shape : The Rio-ipecacuanha is subcylindrical, slender and rather tortous.

Size : Usually 4 to 7 cm. some times upto 18 cm. long and 3 to 5 mm, rarely upto 6 mm thick.

Colour : The surface is dark brown and sometimes has a brick-red appearance owing to adherent earth.

Outer surface : The outer surface is marked by transverse constrictions or fissures which may reach as far as the wood and give an appearance of about eight annulations per centimeter.

Fracture : Short and starchy or horny in the bark, but splintery in the wood.

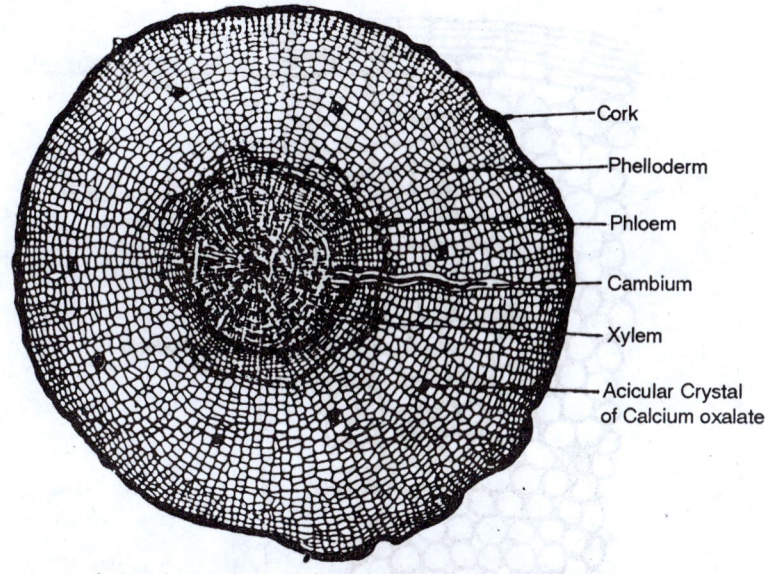

Cork
Phelloderm
Phloem
Cambium
Xylem
Acicular Crystal of Calcium oxalate

Fig. 29 (b) Ipecacuanha Root

The tansversely cut surface shows a central core of yellowish-white dense wood, occupying about one third of the diameter surrounded by the cambium line and a wide greyish bark with a thin brown cork externally. The roots consists on an average of about 80 per cent of starchy bark and 20 per cent of woody core.

The stems which are always present in the drug are recognised by their slender uniform cylindrical shape, about 1 to 3 mm in diameter, by the longitudinally striated surface upon which scars and occasional buds may be found and by the absence of annulations. In the transverse cut surface there is a central pith, about one-sixth of the total diameter, surrounded by a ring of dense yellowish xylem, about 0.75 mm wide, covered externally by a narrow bark. The commercial drug often contains from 3 to 24 percent of stem.

T.S. OF IPECACUANHA ROOT

A transverse section of the root shows the following structures :

1. **Cork :** It consists of a narrow layer of parenchymatous cells.
2. **Phelloderm :** It consists of wide, round parenchyma cells containing starch grains.

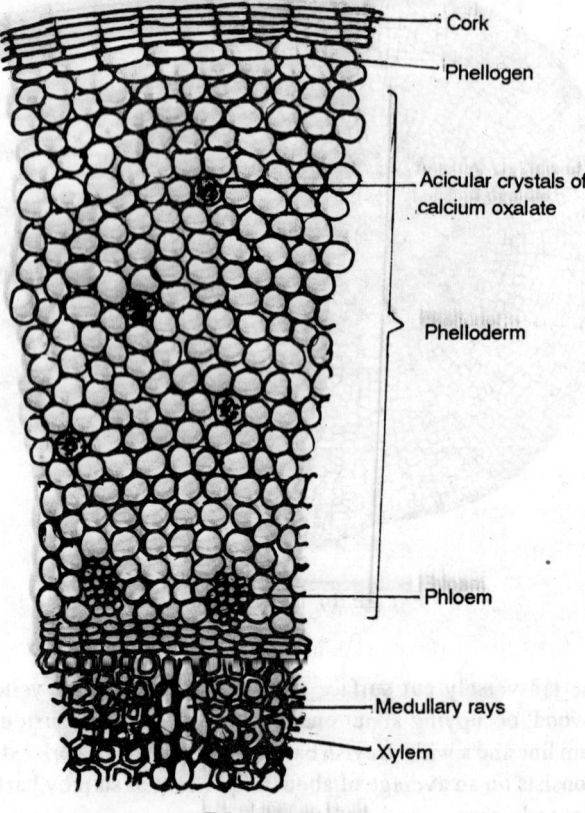

T.S. of Ipecac Root

Fig. 29 (c) Ipecacuanha Root

3. **Secondary phloem :** It consists of a narrow band and a composed of sieve tubes embeded in parenchyma.

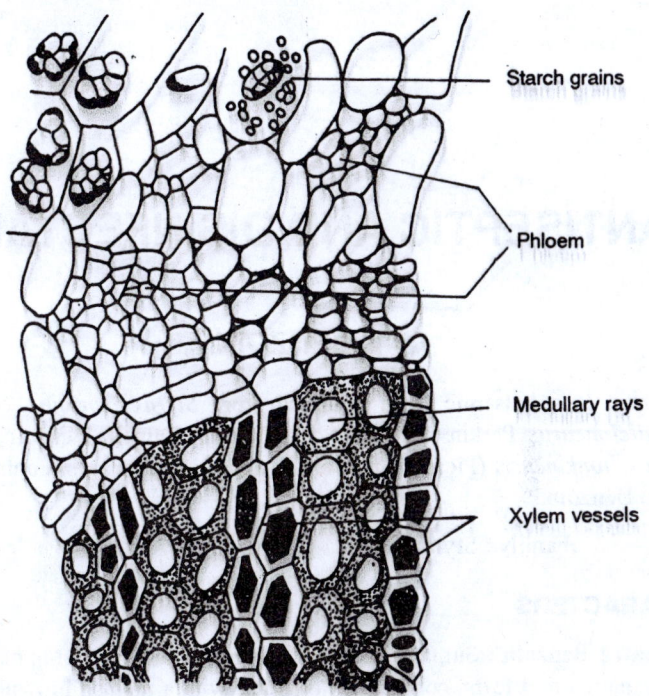

T.S. of Lower part of Root   (Magnified View)

Fig. 29 (d) Ipecacuanha Root

4. **Secondary xylem :** The secondary xylem consists of a narrow tracheidal vessel and tracheids, both having bordered pits.

5. **Xylem paranchyma :** It has simple pits and some of them ore developed as substitute fibres. The cell contains starch grains.

6. **Medullary days :** It consists of 1-2 cell. The cells of medullary rays are wide and may be recognised by the slight radial elongation, of their cells and by their starch content as seen in the sections stained with iodine.

15

ANTISEPTIC AND DISINFECTANTS

1. BENZOIN

Benzoin is a balsamic resin obtained from *Styrax benzoin* or *styrax paralleloneurus* Perkins, known in commerce as Sumatra Benzoin, or from *Styrax tonkinensis* (Pierer) Craib ex Hartwigh, known as in commerce as Siam Benzoin.

Family : Styraceae

CHARACTERS

Sumatra Benzoin : Sumatra Benzoin occurs in blocks or lump of varying size, made up of tears, compacted together, with a reddish brown, reddish grey, or greyish brown resinous mass. The tears are externally yellowish or rusty brown. They are milky white in fresh fracture, hard and brittle at ordinary temperature but softened by heat and becoming gritty on chewing. Its odour resembles that of storax and is not vanilla like. When heated it does not emit a pinaceous odour. When digested with boiling water, the odour suggests cinnamates or storax. Its taste is at first sweetish and then slightly acrid.

Siam Benzoin : Siam Benzoin occurs in pebble like tears of variable size and shape, compressed yellowish brown to rusty brown externally, milky white fracture, separate or very slightly agglutinated, hard and brittle at ordinary temperature but softened by heat and becoming plastic on chewing. It has an agreeable balsamic vanilla-like odour. Its taste is at first sweetish and then slightly acrid.

CHEMICAL TESTS

    (i) To a solution in alcohol add water. The solution becomes milky and the mixture is acid to litmus.

(ii) Heat few pieces in a test tube, a sublimate consisting of plates and small rod-like crystals that strongly polarize light are formed in case of Sumatra Benzoin while a sublimate directly above the melted mass, consisting of numerous long, rod shaped crystals, which do not strongly polarize light are formed in case of Siam Benzoin.

(iii) To 0.25 g of Benzoin add 5 ml of solvent ether and decant 1 ml of the ether solution into a porcelain dish and add to it 2 or 3 drops of sulphuric acid, a deep reddish brown colour is produced in case of Sumatra Benzoin while a deep purplish-red colour is produced in case of Siam Benzoin.

(iv) Heat 0.5 g of Bezoin in a test tube with 10 ml of solution of potassium permanganate; only Sumatra Benzoin develps a strong odour of benzaldehyde.

2. MYRRH

Myrrh is a gum-resin obtained from the stem of *Commiphora molmol* Engier.

Family : Burseraceae

CHARACTERS

Form : It occurs in irregular rounded tears.

Size : About 2.5 cm in diameter or in masses of agglutinated tears, sometimes as much as 10 cm. across.

Colour : It is reddish-brown with a rough, dull and dusty surface.

Texture : Brittle

Fracture : Breaks with granular fracture.

Fractured surface : The fractured surface is unctuous and often marked by whitish spots or veins. Thin splinters are transluscent or almost transparent.

Odour : It has an agreeable aromatic odour.

Taste : It has bitter and acrid, but not unpleasant taste.

CHEMICAL TEST

(i) When triturated with water it form a yellowish emulsion.

(ii) Extract small quantity of powdered Myrrh with ether and evaporate the solvent in such a way that a thin film of the resin is left in the dish. Pass the vapour of bromine or fumes of nitric acid over the film. A deep violet colour is produced.

3. NIM

Nim or Neem is obtained from *Azadirachta indica* A Juis (Synonym *Melia Indica*).

Family : Meliaceae

MORPHOLOGICAL CHARACTERS

Leaves :

Leaves are compound, alternate, exstipulate 28-30 cm long with swollen base leaflets are short stalked, ovate lanceolate with serrate margin and glossy surface. Young leaves are reddish green while mature one are dark green.

Flower

Inflorescence is long slender, axillary with abundant flowers.

Flowers are pale yellow as white with characteristic smell and bisexual calyx is imbricate or valvate with 3-5 sepals Corolla is oblong spreading and spatulate.

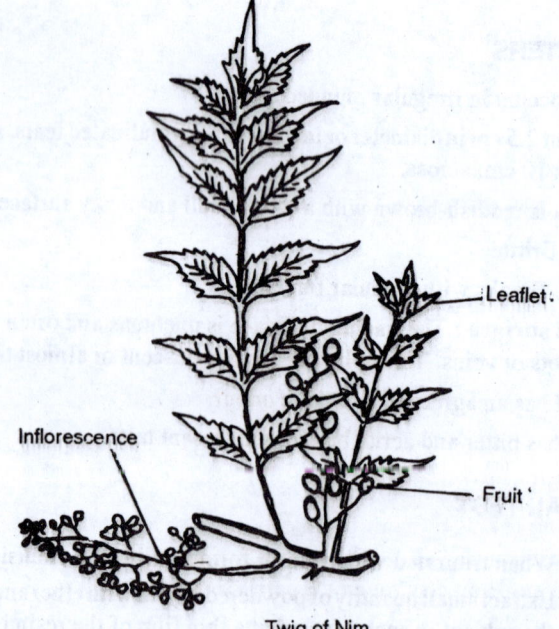

Twig of Nim

Fig. 30. Nim

Androcium consist of 10 stamers.

Gynoecium is tricarpellary, syncarpous ovary is superior, trilocular at the base and unilocular above with parietal placentation.

4. CURCUMA
(Turmeric)

Turmeric consists of the prepared rhizomes of *Curcuma domestica*. Valeton.

Family : Zingiberaceae

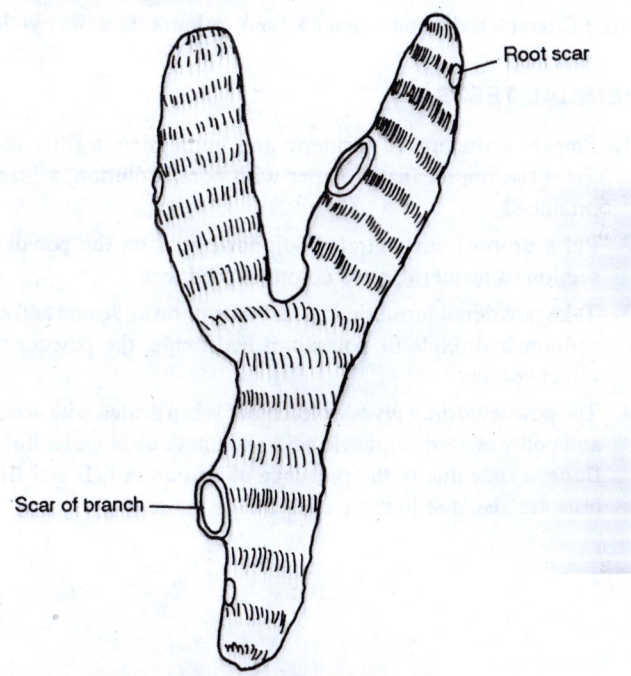

Fig. 31. Turmeric

Morphological Characters

Shape : Finger or long turmeric occurs in curved or nearly straight cylindrical pieces bluntly tapering at each end. The primary rhizomes are pear shaped or ovate and are known as round turmeric or bulb.

Size : Long turmeric is 4-7 cm long and 1-1.5 cm wide.

Colour : The outer surface is deep yellowish brown.

Outer surface : The outer surface is longitudinally wrinkled and marked with transverse rings (leaf-scars).

Fracture : Short, internally they have a uniform dull brownish-yellow appearance and tough horny consistence.

The smoothed transverse surface exhibits a paler ring separating the stele from the cortex.

The bulb or round turmeric very much resembles the long turmeric, but as its name indicates, shorter and thicker.

Odour : The drug has characteristic odour.

Taste : Characteristic and when chewed, colours the saliva yellow.

CHEMICAL TESTS

1. Prepare a tincture of turmeric and impregnate a filter paper with it. Treat the impreganated paper with borax solution, a green colour is produced.

2. Put a drop of concentrated sulphuric acid on the powder or a thick section of turmeric, a red colour is produced.

3. Take powdered turmeric in a test tube or on slide and add a solution of sodium hydroxide or potassium hydroxide, the powder gives red to violet colour.

4. The powdered drug gives violet colour when treated with acetic anhydride and concentrated sulphuric acid and under ultra violet light shows red fluorescence due to the presence of curcumin I, II and III. The other tests are also due to these constituents.

16

ANTIMALARIALS

CINCHONA

Cinchona is the dried bark of *Cinchona calisaya*, *C. ledgeriana*, *C. officinalis* and *C. succirubra*.

Family : Rubiaceae

CINCHONA

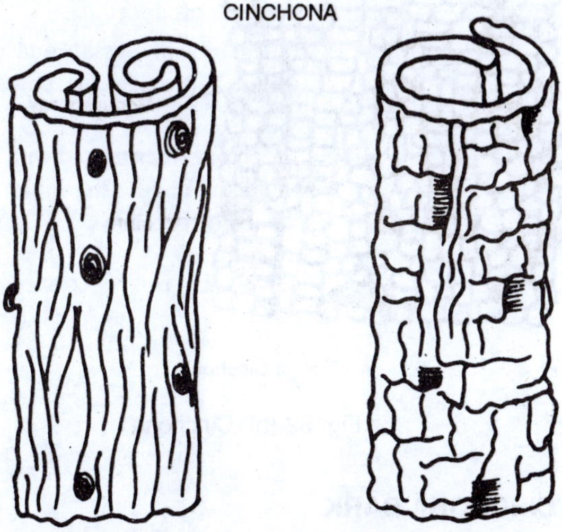

Red Cinchona (Double quill)   Calisaya Bark (Single quill)

Fig. 32 (a) The Bark

Morphological Characters

Shape : Curved, quill and double quill.

Size : 30 cm long, 1.5 to 2 cm in diameter, 2 to 8 mm. thick.

Colour : Reddish brown to yellowish brown.

Outer surface : Rough, longitudinal, transverse cracks or fissures, ridges and protuberances. Greyish patches of moss or lichens are present.

Fracture : Short in outer bark and fibrous in inner part.

Odour : Distinct and characteristic

Taste : Bitter

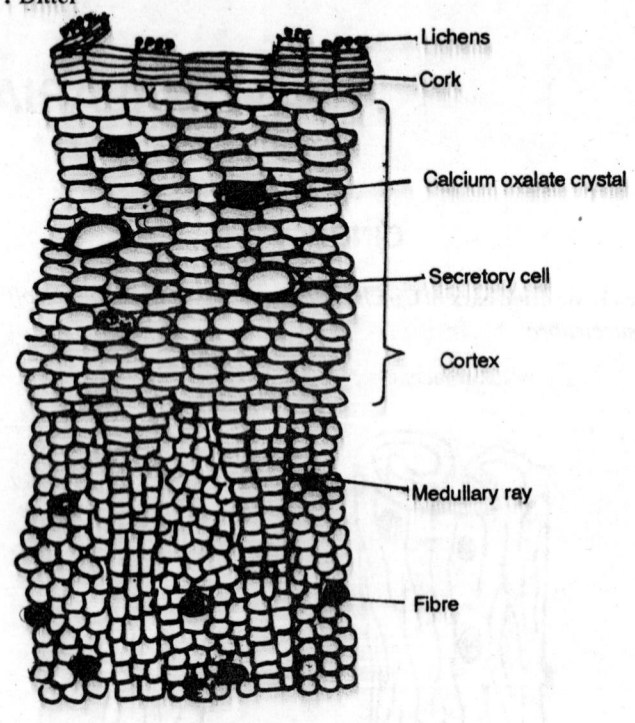

T.S. of Cinchona

Fig. 32 (b) Cinchona

T.S. OF CINCHONA BARK

It shows the following structures

Cork : Numerous layers of thin walled, flat polygonal cells filled with reddish brown mass. Cork is occassionally covered with lichens.

Cortex : It is narrow, parenchymatous. Cells contain starch grains and microcrystals of calcium oxalate. Secretion canals are also present.

Phloem fibres : Lignified phloem fibres with tubular fennel shaped pits.

Pholem parenchyma : Consist of cells with thin, dark reddish brown walls, some containing microprisms of calcium oxalate.

Medullary rays (Medullary) : They are from one to three seriate Sclereids are absent

OXYTOCICS

ERGOT

The drug is the dried sclerotium of *Claviceps purpurea* (Fries) Tulsane.

Family : Clavicipitaceae

It develops on plants of rye, *Secale cereale*.

Family : Graminae

At present the ergot alkaloids are also produced from the fermentation broth in which mycelium of selected strains of claviceps are grown in submerged cultures.

Morphological Characters

Shape : The sclerotium is fusiform in shape and is usually slightly curved.

Size : It is 1 to 4 cm long and 2 to 7 mm broad.

Outer surface : The outer surface is dark violet black in colour which is longitudinally furrowed with occasional small transverse cracks.

Fractrue : The drug breaks with short fracture.

Fractured surface : White or pinkish white zone of pseudoparenchyma. Dark lines radiating from the centre are also visible.

Odour . Ergot has a characteristic odour.

Taste : Unpleasant

CHEMICAL TESTS

(i) Treat the powdered ergot with sodium hydroxide solution, a smell of trimethylamine is produced.

(ii) On exposing ergot to filtered ultra violet light a red florescence is seen.

(iii) Extract powdered ergot with chloroform in presence of sodium carbonate. To chloroform extract add 2 ml of a reagent consisting of 0.1 g of p dimethylaminobenzaldehyde, 100 ml 35% v/v sulphuric acid and 1.5 ml of 5% ferric chloride. A deep blue colour is produced. This test is due to ergotoxine.

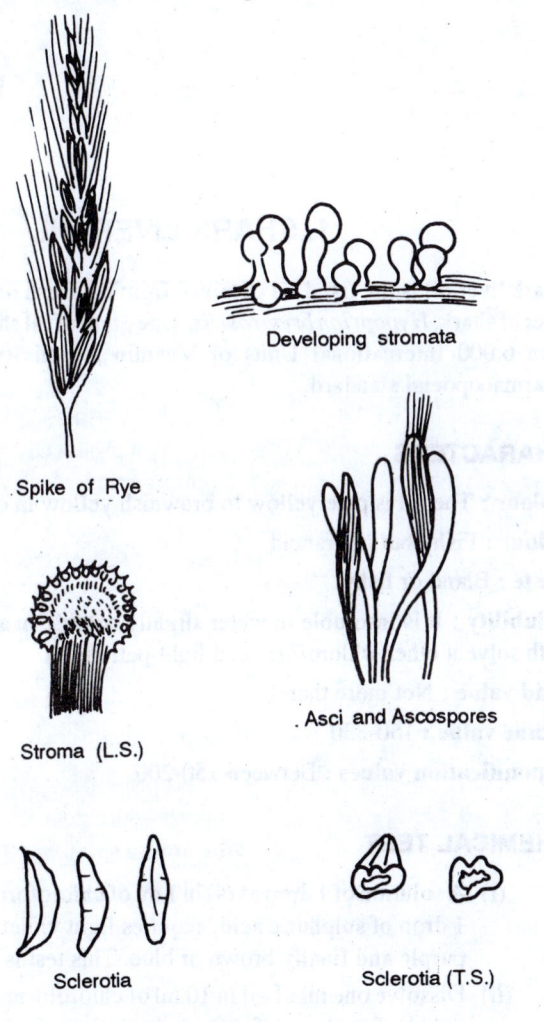

Spike of Rye

Developing stromata

Stroma (L.S.)

Asci and Ascospores

Sclerotia

Sclerotia (T.S.)

Fig. 33. Ergot

VITAMINS

1. SHARK LIVER OIL

Shark liver oil is the fixed oil obtained from the fresh or carefully preserved liver of shark, *Hypoprion brevirostris*. One gram of oil should contain not less than 6,000 International Units of Vitamin A activity as per the Indian Pharmacopoeial standard.

CHARACTERS

Colour : The oil is pale yellow to brownish yellow in colour.

Odour : Fishy but not rancid

Taste : Bland or fishy

Solubility : It is insoluble in water slightly soluble in alcohol and miscible with solvent ether, chloroform and light-petroleum.

Acid value : Not more than 2

Iodine value : 160-350

Saponification values : Between 150-200

CHEMICAL TEST

(i) A solution of 1 drop of oil in 1 ml of chloroform, when shaken with 1 drop of sulphuric acid, acquires light violet colour, changing to purple and finally brown or blue. This test is due to vitamin A.

(ii) Dissolve one ml of oil in 10 ml of chloroform in a dry test tube. To it add a few drops of saturated solution of antimony trichloride in chloroform, a blue colour is produced. This test is also due to the presence of vitamin A.

2. AMLA

The drug consists of the fresh or dried fruit of *Emblica officinalis*   L or *Phyllanthus embelica* Linn.

Family : Euphorbiaceae

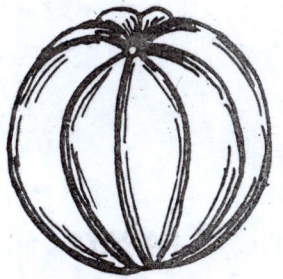

Fig. 34 Amla

CHARACTERS

The fruit is a tricarpellary drupe with fleshy mesocarp and stony endocarp.

Shape : Globose

Colour : Green when unripe but turns yellow on maturity.

Outer surface : The outer surface of the fruit is smooth shiny having six verticle furrows. A minute depression left after removal of the peduncle is distinctly observed at one end of the fruit.

Taste : Sour and astringent.

ENZYMES

1. PAPAYA

It is the unripe Fruit of *Carica papaya* Linn. belonging to family caricaceae.

GENERAL MORPHOLOGY OF PLANT AND FRUIT

Plant of papaya attains a height of 5-6 meters. The fruit is about 30 cm in length and weight varies according to the size of fruit with maximum of 5 kg. The epicarp adheres to the orange coloured fleshy sarcocarp, which surrounds the central cavity. The cavity contains numerous black seeds which are round in shape.

Papain : This term is used for both crude dried latex obtained from unripe fruit and crystalline proteolytic enzyme obtained from it.

Characters of Papain : It is white or greyish white slightly hygroscopic powder.

Solubility : It is incompletely soluble in water or glycerol and insoluble in most of the organic solvents.

Potency : It varies according to the process of preparation, but usual grade digests 35 times its own weight of lean meat.

2. DIASTASE

It is an amylolytic enzyme. It is of two types.

(a) **Salivary Diastase :** It is also called animal diastase found in the digestive tract of animals.

(b) **Malt Diastase :** It is formed during the germination of barley grains.

CHARACTERS

Colour: It is yellowish white amorphous powder occurs as translucent scales.

Solubility : It is soluble in water with slight turbidity. It is insoluble in alcohol.

Activity : It converts 50 times its own weight of potato starch into sugar (dextrin and maltose) in 30 minutes. It has maximum activity at neutral pH.

3. YEAST

Yeast is the dried unicellular fungi obtained from *Saccharomyces cerevisiae* and *S. caresbergensis*.

Family : Saccharomycetaceae

CHARACTERS

It occurs a powder or flakes.

Colour : It has buff or brownish buff colour.

Odour : It has characteristic odour.

Taste : Varies according to the source and method of preparation.

PERFUMES AND FLAVOURING AGENTS

1. PEPPERMINT OIL

Peppermint oil is obtained from the aerial parts of *Mentha piperita* Linn.

Family : Labiatae

CHARACTERS OF THE PLANT

It is a herbaceous perennial plant with a creeping rhizome.

Stem : The stem is erect, square and smooth.

Leaves : Leaves are opposite and decussate, shortly petiolate (Petiole 0.5 to 1 cm. long), nearly glabrous, ovate, about 3 to 8 cm long and twice as long as broad, margin serrate and apex acute.

Inflorescence : It is in ovoid-cylindrical terminal heads and is interrupted below.

Flowers : They have the floral formula

$K_{(5)}$ $C_{(5)}$ $A_{(4)}$ equal $G_{(2)}$, 4 loculi with one ovule in each.

Corolla campanulate, only a little longer than the calyx, 4 or 5 cleft with nearly equal lobes, *throat* of the corolla almost smooth, calyx throat naked, teeth hispid, base of calyx and pedicel smooth

Fruit : 4, nutlets.

The stem of the black variety are reddish purple and its leaves are dark green, whereas the true or white variety is more green.

Odour : Strong aromatic

Taste : Pungent and cooling.

Character of oil : It is a colourless yellowish liquid.

Odour : Characteristic and pleasant

Taste : Pungent followed by a cooling sensation.

Solubility : 1 ml of oil dissolves in 3.5-4.0 ml of 70% alcohol.

Weight per ml : 0.89 - 0.919 g. at 25°

Optical rotation : -18° to -33° at 25°.

2. LEMON OIL

Lemon oil is the volatile oil expressed from fresh lemon peel. It contains not less than 4 percent w/w of aldehyde, calculated as citral, $C_{10}H_{16}O$. The lemon peel is obtained from the fruits of *Citrus limon* (L) Burm.

> Family : Rutaceae

CHARACTERS

Colour : The oil is a pale yellow or greenish yellow liquid.

Odour : Lemon like.

Taste : Warm and slightly bitter.

Solubility : Souble in 3 parts of alcohol.

Optical rotation : +57° to +65°

Refractive index : 1.4711 to 1.4761 at 25°C.

Wt. per ml : 0.849 to 0.855 g at 25°C.

Non volatile matter : Evaporate 5 g in a flat bottomed nickel dish, 9 cm in diameter and 1.5 cm in depth, by heating on a vigorously boiling water-bath for a total of four hours; the residue weighs not less than 75 mg and not more than 150 mg.

3. ORANGE OIL

The orange oil is obtained from the fresh or dried orange peel of the fruit of *Citrus chrysocarpa Lush* (*Citrus aurantium* Linn).

> Family : Rutaceae

CHARACTERS OF DRIED ORANGE PEEL

The dried orange peel consists of thin strips with little of inner dirty white portion of the rind. Oil glands are visible on the surface of the peel as small dots of dark orange colour. The peel has short fracture; sweet fragrant odour and bitter aromatic taste.

CHARACTERS OF FRESH ORANGE PEEL

The fresh orange peel consists of thin strips with little of the inner white portion of the rind, 3-4 cm thick the outer surface is orange red in colour, glabrous, smooth, glossy, oily and slightly pitted. There are visible oil glands as small dots of dark orange colour.

Odour and taste is similar to dried orange peel.

4. LEMON-GRASS OIL

Lemon grass oil is the volatile oil distilled from *Cymbopogon flexuous* stapf.

Family : Graminae

It contain not less than 75 percent w/w of aldehye, calculated as citrat, $C_{10}H_{16}O$.

CHARACTERS

The oil is reddish yellow to brown. It has an odour of lemon oil.

Solubility : Almost entirely soluble in 3 parts of alcohol.

Wt. per ml : 0.829 to 0.909 at 25°C.

Optical rotation : -3° to +1°

Refractive index : 1.4808 to 1.4868. at 25°C.

5. SANDAL WOOD OIL

Sandal wood is obtained from *Santalum album* Linn.

Family : Santalaceae

CHARACTERS

In sandal, sapwood and heartwood are clearly demarcated. The root is also scented so harvesting is done by uprooting. Heart wood formation occurs when the tree is about 20 year old tree. A tree of 100 cm girth yields 88 kg of sandal wood. Odour of wood is characteristic aromatic.

Characterstic of the oil : It is oily viscous liquid.

Colour and appearance : Nearly colourless to golden yellow.

Odour : Pleasant, sweet woody and persistent.

Specific gravity at 30° : 0.962 - 0.76

Rotation : -15 to -20

Refractive index at 30° : 1.499 - 1.506

Esters (Calculated as santalyl acetates) : 20 %

Free alcohols (calculated as sandal oil% by weight) : 90%

21

PHARMACEUTICAL AIDS

1. HONEY

Honey is a saccharine fluid made by the honey-bees, *Apis mellifera* Linn, order Hymenoptera from the nectar of various flowers.

Family : Apidae.

Characters : Honey is a viscous, clear transluscent liquid.

Colour : Yellowish or yellowish brown. It becomes partially crystalline.

Solubility : Honey is soluble in water. it is insoluble in alcohol and other organic solvent.

Optical activity : Honey is optically active with rotation between +0.6 to 0.3.

CHEMICAL TESTS

(i) The weight per ml of honey is between 1.35 to 1.37 g.

(ii) Prepare a solution of honey by dissolving one part of the drug in five parts of water.

   (a) To one ml of the above solution of honey, add one ml of Fehling's solution and warm on a water bath. The colour of the Fehling's solution gets reduced. On further heating brick red precipitate is formed due to reducing sugars present in the drug.

   (b) To 5 ml of the above solution of honey, add 2.5 ml of diethyl ether shake the solution. Separate the ether layer and transfer it to an evaporating china dish. Evaporate ether completely and to the residue add one drop of 1% w/v solution of resorcinol in concentrated hydrochloric acid. Pure honey should not give cherry red colour. But if honey is adulterated with artificial invert sugar red colour will develop because the artificial invert sugar contains furfural, which gives red colour with resorcinol in hydrochloric acid.

2. ARACHIS OIL
(Groundnut oil, Peanut oil)

Arachis oil is the fixed oil obtained from the seed kernels of *Arachis hypogea* Linn.

Family : Leguminosae

CHARACTERS

Colour : Colourless to pale yellow liquid

Odour : Ground nut like

Taste : Bland

It is a non drying oil and on long exposure to air it becomes rancid. The authentic oil has following constant values.

(a) Acid value : Not more than 2

(b) Iodine value : 85-100

(c) Saponification value : 185-195

(d) Refractive index : 1.4678 - 1.4608.

The oil is lighter than water.

3. STARCH

Starch of pharmaceutical use consists of the grain separated from tubers of potato, *Solanum tuberosum* L.Family : Solanaceae or from the mature grains of maize, *Zea mays* L or from the mature grains of wheat *Triticum aestivum* L. or the grains of rice, *Oryza sativa* L.

Family : Graminae

Morphological Characters of Commercial Starch

Starch	Colour	Shape	Size	Striation	Hilum	Form
1.Potato	light yellow colour	Flattened ovoid or subspherical	30-70 100 μ round grain are 10-35 μ in diameter	Striation are well marked	The hilum is a point at the narrow end of the grain and is called eccentric hilum	Single as well as compound

(Contd.)

Starch	Colour	Shape	Size	Striation	Hilum	Form
2. Maize	White grains	Uniform shape Polyhedral with blunt angles or less round	5-20 μ in diameter	Striation are seen in the larger grain	In the centre the hilum is in the form of a cleft with two or three radiatting lines	Single as well compound grain
3. Wheat	Cream coloured	Lenticular	15-50 μ in diameter		Hilum present as a small point in the centre	
4. Rice	White	Minutes polyhedral grains with sharp angles	3-6 μ in diameter	Not visible	Very small present in the centre	Compound grain, a few single

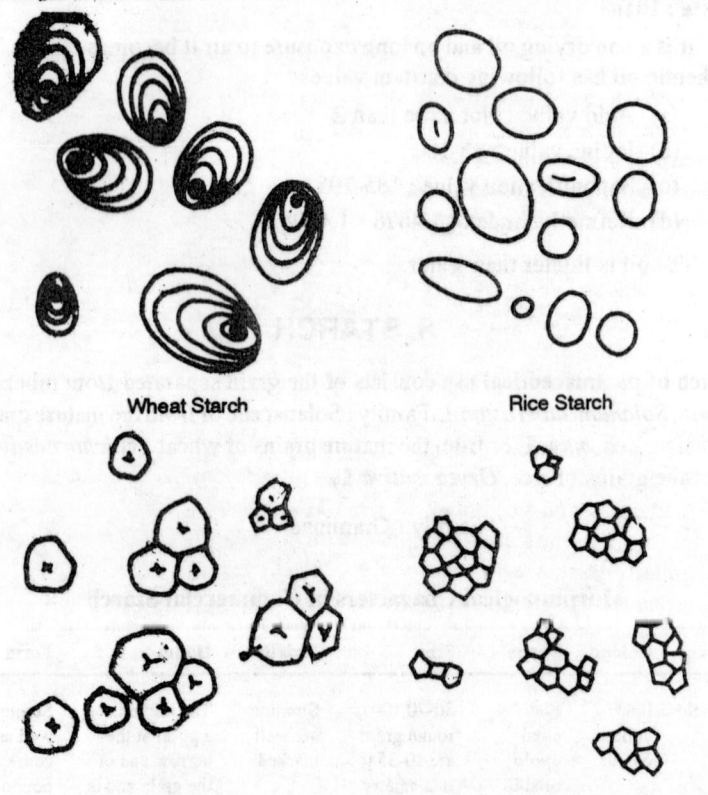

Wheat Starch   Rice Starch

Potato starch   Maize starch

Fig. 35. Starches

CHEMICAL TESTS

(i) If one g of starch is boiled will 15 ml water for two minutes and cooled, a transluscent viscous jelly is formed.

(ii) To a portion of the above jelly add a drop of dilute Iodine solution. Immediate blue colour is produced. The blue colour disappears on warming and appears again on cooling.

4. KAOLIN

Kaolin is a pure variety of clay produced by weathering and decomposition of the feldspar of granite.

CHARACTERS

Kolin is a very fine clay, crumbling to powder when pressed between the fingers and having a slightly soapy feel. It is white or white with a faint yellowish tint, it has a density of 2.3 and is insoluble in water. Dilute acids and alkalies do not affect kaolin, but strong hydrochloric acids decomposes it partially and prolonged heating with strong sulphuric acid converts it partially into insoluble silica and sulphate of aluminium. When dry it is odourless, but develops a clay like odour when moistened. It has a slight earthy taste.

By subjecting crude kaolin to the process of elutriation, various grades are produced, differing in the size of the particle, present. The variety containing the smallest particles is largely colloidal in nature and this type used for internal administration. A coarser variety containing no colloidal matter is used for assisting filtration and for making preparatious such as Kaolin Poultice.

The two varietis can be distinguished by their behaviour towards water. The colloidal type, when knead with a small amount of water, forms a stiff, sticky mass, and when suspended in water a permanent turbid fluid results and only a part of the Kaolin is deposited on the bottom. The coarser Kaolin when similarly treated with water yields a plastic but less sticky mass, and when suspended in water the whole of this coarser kaolin eventually settles, leaving a clear supernatant liquid.

5. PECTIN

It is a complex purified carbohydrate obtained from the dilute acid extract of the peel of citrus fruits such as *Citrus limon* or *C. aurantium* L.

Family : Rutaceae

Besides citrus fruits pulp of apple, papaya, guava and mangoes is also rich source of pectin.

CHARACTERS

It occurs in the form of coarse or fine powder.

Colour : Cream

Odour : None

Solubility : It is completely soluble in 20 parts of water and the solution is colloidal, viscous and acidic to litmus paper. It is insoluble is alcohol and other organic solvents. With 9 parts of water, it form a jelly if heated. It is stable in acidic medium.

CHEMICAL TESTS

1. Take 1 g of pectin in a test tube and add 9 ml of water and heat gently, it forms a stiff jelly.
2. Prepare 1 % solution of pectin. To 5 ml of this solution add one ml of 2% aqueous solution of sodium hydroxide. Within 20 minutes a transparent gel is formed. When this gel is shaken with dilute hydrochloric acid, gelatinous precipitates are formed which on boiling become white.

6. OLIVE OIL

Olive oil is the oil expressed from the pericarp of the ripe fruits of the olive tree, *Olea europoea* Linn.

Family : Oleaceae

The medicinal oil is also called as virgin oil.

CHARACTERS

Colour : It is a pale yellow or greenish yellow coloured liquid.

Odour : Characteristic

Taste : Bland taste

It is a liquid at ordinary temperature but when cooled at 10°C it assumes a pasty consistency, form deposition of solid fats and at 0°C it becomes nearly solid, granular mass.

Specific gravity : 0.915 to 0.918

Acid value : Not more than 1

Iodine value: 79 to 87

Refractive index : 1.4605 to 1.4635 at 40°C.

The olive oil is adultrated with cotton seed oil or with sesame oil or with arachis oil. These oil can be detected in olive oil by the following chemical tests.

(i) For detection of cotton seed oil the following two tests may be performed.

Halphen's test : Warm 2 ml of oil with 1 ml of amyl alcohol and 1 ml of 1 percent solution of sulphur in carbon disulphide for ten minutes on a water bath. No red colour should be developed, but this test is positive i.e. red colour is produced if cotton seed oil is present in the sample.

(ii) For detection of sesame oil, the following test is performed.

2 ml of the oil is mixed with 1 ml of hydrochloric acid containing 1 per cent sucrose. The solution is shaken for 1 minute, no pink colour should appear. If sesame oil is present in the oil pink colour will appear in the solution.

(iii) For detection of Arachis oil : The Arachis oil is detected by separating the fatty acids, purifying them and taking their melting point, which should not be higher than 71°C. Arachidic acid which is present in Arachis oil has a melting point of 77°C.

7. LANOLIN
(Wool fat)

Lanolin is the purified, faltty substance prepared from the wool of the sheep, *Ovis aries.*

Family : Bovidae

It contains 25-30% water and hence called as hydrous wool fat. Puried wool fat is anhydrous lanolin.

CHARACTERS

Form : Purified wool fat is a tenacious, unctuous solid.

Colour : Yellow

Odour : Characteristic

Taste : Bland taste

Melting point : 34° to 40°C

Solubility : It is soluble in acetone, benzene and other organic solvents but it is insoluble in water.

Saponificatian value : 94 - 106

Iodine value : 18-32

CHEMICAL TEST

(i) Disolve 0.5 g of lanolin in 5 ml of chloroform, add 1 ml of acetic anhydride and 2 drops of sulphuric acid, a deep green colour is produced due to the presence of cholesterol.

8. BEES-WAX

Bees-wax is obtained from the honey comb of the bee, *Apis mellifera* L. and other species of Apis.

Family : Apidae

The wax is secreted by the worker bee in the last four segments of the abdomen and excreted through the pores. The young worker bees utilize the wax in the construction of the comb.

CHARACTERS

Form : It is a solid non crystalline substance. Breaks with granular fracture.

Colour : Yellow or brownish yellow

Odour : Agreeable honey like

Melting poinl : 60-65°C

Specific gravity : 0.958 to 0.970 lighter than water

Refractive index : 1.4380 to 1.4420

Acid value : 17-23

Ester value : 70-80

Solubility : It is insoluble in water. It is readily soluble in hot oil of turpentine but is partially and sparingly soluble in alcohol, soluble in warm ether, chloroform and in fixed oils and volatile oils.

9. ACACIA

Acacia gum is dried exudation from its stem and branches of *Acacia senegal* willdew and other species of Acacia.

Family : Leguminosae

CHARACTERS

Form : It occurs in rounded or ovoid tears, brittle in nature.

Size : About 0.5 to 4 or sometimes as much as 6 cm in diameter.

Colour : White, but sometimes show a yellowish tinge. The tears are opaque due to the presence in the outer part of the tears of small numerous fissures. Inferior grades are yellow or reddish brown in colour and contain traces of tannin.

Solubility : It is insoluble in alcohol, but dissolve freely in water forming a translucent, viscid liquid.

Optical activity : 10% solution is laevo-rotatory.

CHEMICAL TESTS

(i) Mount a small quantity of powder in ruthenium red solution and examine in microscope. The particles do not get red colour (distinction from agar).

(ii) To 5 ml of 2% w/v solution, add 1 ml of strong lead subacetate solution, A flocculent white precipitate is produced.

(iii) Dissolve 0.25 g in 5 ml of water by shaking in cold, add 0.5 ml of hydrogen peroxide solution and 0.5 ml of 1% solution of benzidine in alcohol. Shake and allow to stand. A deep blue colour which is unstable is noticed, due to the enzyme oxidase.

(iv) To 10 ml of a 2% w/v solution, add 0.2 ml of a 20% w/v solution of lead acetate. No precipitate is produced (distinction from agar and tragacanth)

(v) To 0.1 g of powder, add 1 ml of N/50 iodine. The mixture does not acquire crimson colour. (distinction from agar and tragacanth).

(vi) To 1 ml of solution, add 4 ml of water and dilute hydrochloric acid and boil for a few minutes. Hydrolysis takes place and reducing sugars are produced. Add Fehling's solution and heat, red precipitate of cuprous oxide is produced.

10. TRAGACANTH

Tragacanth gum is a dried gumny exudation from the stem of *Astragalus gummifer* lab.

Family : Leguminosae

Indian tragacanth is obtained from *Sterculia urens* Roxburgh.

Family : Sterculiaceae

CHARACTERS

Form : It occurs in thin, flattened, curved, ribbon-shaped flakes of translucent, horny appearance.

Colour : Colourless or faint yellow.

Size : The flakes are often 3 cm long 1 cm wide and about 2 mm thick.

Outer surface : The outer surface is marked with numerous concentric longitudinal and transverse ridges.

Fracture : Short

Odour: None

Taste : Tasteless

If soaked in water, it swells considerably forming a tenacious gelatinous mass, but only 8-10% dissolves.

CHEMICAL TESTS

1. To 4 ml of a 0.5 % w/v solution add 0.5 ml of hydrochloric acid and heat for 30 minutes on a water bath. Divide the liquid into two parts.

    (a) To one part, add 1.5 ml of sodium hydroxide solution and Fehling's solution, warm on water bath, red precipitate is produced.

    (b) To the second part, add barium chloride solution (10%). No precipitate is obtained (distinction from agar).

2. To a 0.5% w/v solution of the gum, add 20% w/v solution of lead acetate. A voluminous flocculent precipitate is obtained (distinction from acacia).

3. Mount a small quantity of powder in ruthenium red and examine. microscopically, particles do not acquire pink colour (distinction from indian tragacanth).

4. To 0.1 g of powder, add N/50 iodine the mixture acquires an olive green colour (distinction from acacia and agar).

5. Warm the powder with 5% aqueous caustic potash. Canary yellow colour is produced.

11. SODIUM ALGINATE

Alginates are prepared from several species of the class Phaeophyceae or brown algae. The most importent are species of *Laminaria* known as kelps or sea tangles, and species of Fucus, known as wracks. Sodium alginate is prepared by beating the seaweeds with solution of calcium chloride when the calcium alginates are precipitated.

CHARACTERS

Sodium alginate is a white or slightly yellowish powder, freely soluble in hot or cold water, a 4 percent solution giving a thick viscous liquid. The solution is not coagulated by heat and does not set to a jelly on cooling, it can, however, be made to gel by converting it partly into a calcium salt by adding a small proportion of calcium chloride.

CHEMICAL TEST

Alginic acid is a polyuronic acid. It does not reduce Fehling's solution, but after hydrolysis with sulphuric acid or hydrochloric acid the product reduces Fehling's solution rapidly.

12. AGAR

Agar is the bleached and dried product obtained by concentrating a decoction made from vrious species of algae belonging to the class Rhodophyceae. Agar from Japan is made chiefly from species of *Gelidium,* specially *G. elegans* kutz., *G. amansii kutz., G. polycladum* Sond.

Family : Gelidiaceae

CHARACTERS

Form : It occurs is translucent strips. Occasionally in flattened sticks, also as coarse powder.

Size : Each strip is about 60 cm by 0.5 to 1.0 cm and 0.1 mm thick. The flattened sticks are about 30 cm long by 2.5 cm wide and 5-7 mm thick.

Colour : Slightly yellow tent.

Surface : The surface is wrinkled and somewhat micaceous and various species of diatoms are found embeded in it, the most characteristic being species of *Arachnoidiscus* which is discoid and has a sculpturing on its valves in the form of radiating lines and concentric circles, producing a resemblance to a spider's web.

Texture : Agar is tough and difficult to break.

Odour : Slight

Taste : Faintly salty mucilaginous taste

SOLUBILITY

(i) It swells in cold water but only a small fraction dissolves.

(ii) 1% solution may be made by boiling. On cooling, it forms a hard jelly.

CHEMICAL TESTS

(i) With ruthenium red the powdered agar gives red colour when examined under microscope.

(ii) When N/50 iodine solution is added to the powder, it produces crimson to brown colour.

(iii) Add 0.5 ml of dilute hydrochloric acid to 0.5% aqueous solution of drug and heat on water bath for 30 minutes, divide the solution in two parts.

    (a) Add to one part 3 ml of 10% caustic soda solution and 2 ml of Fehling's solution and heat on water bath. Reduction takes place due to galactose.

    (b) To the second part add barium chloride solution (10%), white precipitate of barium sulphate is obtained.

(iii) Agar is incinerated to ash, dilute hydrochloric acid added and observed under microscope. Skeletons and sponge spicules of diatoms are seen.

The following tests are negative because Agar does not contain nitrogen.

(i) Heating with soda lime, ammonia is not produced.

(ii) With Millon's reagent it does not give any precipitate.

(iii) When treated will tannic acid, no precipitate is produced.

13. GUAR GUM

Gaur gum is the powder of endosperm of the seeds of *Cyamopsis tetragonolobus* Linn and other species of Cyamopsis.

    Family : *Leguminosae*

CHARACTERS

The gum is almost colourless or pale yellowish white powder. It has characteristic odour and taste. When examined in lactophenol mount under microscope, it shows irregular particles of angular shape and various sizes. In water it swells rapidly forming a translucent suspension.

SOLUBILITY

When the gum is stirred with 50 parts of water, a thick jelly is formed which with further addition of 150 parts of water, yields a thick transparent suspension. It is insoluble in alcohol.

CHEMICAL TESTS

1. To 0.1 g of gum add 1 ml of 0.2 N iodine. The mixture does not aquire olive green colour.

2. Dissolve 0.1 of gum in 20 ml of water by shaking and add 0.5 ml hydrogen peroxide solution add 0.5 ml of 1% w/v solution of benzidine in 90% alcohol shake and allow to stand. No blue colour is produced (distinction from gum acacia).

3. Mount a small quantity of gum in solution of ruthenium red and examine under microscope. Particle do not acquire pink colour. (distinction from sterculia gum and agar).

4. To 0.5% w/v solution of gum add 20% w/v solution of lead acetate, a flocculant precipitate is produced (distinction from acacia and sterculia gum).

5. A 0.5% w/v solution of gum is neutral to litmus.

6. Foreign organic matter is not more than 0.5%.

7. Ash value : note more than 0.5%.

8. Loss on drying : Loss is not more than 8% of its weight when dried to constant weight at 105°C.

14. GELATIN

Gelatin is a protein derivative obtained by evaporating an aqueous extract made from skins, tendons and bones derived from various domestic animals, such as the Ox, *Bos taurus* Linn, the sheep, *Ovis aries* Linn.

Family : Bovidae

Order : Ungulata

Class : Mammalia

CHARACTERS

Form : It occurs in thin sheets, or in shreds or in powder form.

Colour : It is nearly colourless or pale yellow

Odour : None

Fracture : When broken it at first bends and then breaks suddenly with a short fracture

Taste : Tasteless

SOLUBILITY

(i) In cold water it swells and when heated dissolves

(ii) It is soluble in acetic acid and glycerine

(iii) It is Insoluble in alcohol and ether.

Other characters : Gelatin yields 0.6 2 percent of ash. It contains 12-17 per cent of moisture.

CHEMICAL TESTS

(i) Make 2 percent of the aqueous solution of gelatin by heating. On cooling it form a jelly. The gelatinising property is destroyed by boiling for long time.

(ii) To a aqueous soluion of gelatin add a drop of picric acid or tannic acid solution, a precipitate is produced. The precipitate is formed due to the formation of protein picrate or protein tannate.

(iii) Heat gelatin with soda lime in a test tube. Fumes of ammonia evolves indicating the presence of proteins. This test is negative with agar.

(iv) To an aqueous solution of gelatin add few drops of mercuric nitrate solution, a white precipitate is formed. Heat the test tube, the precipitate becomes brick-red in colour.

(v) When gelatin is treated with formaldehyde or potassium dichromate, and exposed to light, it becomes insoluble.

MISCELLANEOUS

1. LIQUORICE

Glycyrrhiza root consists of the stolons and roots of various species of Glycyrrhiza i.e. *Glycyrrhiza glabra* Linn or *G. glandulifera wald* or *G. violacea*

Family : Leguminosae

Morphological Characters

Shape : The unpeeled pieces of the root ore unbranched, straight unbranched and cylindrical peeled pieces are angular.

Size : The roots are upto 1 meter in length and are 1 to 2 cm in diameter. Sometime they also occur in small pieces of about 20 cm.

Colour : The outer surface is dark reddish brown. Peeled liquorice is yellow in colour.

Outer surface : The outer surface show longitudinal wrinkles and the stolen bears occasional small buds, scale leaves and scars of slender side roots.

Fracture : The fracture is fibrous in the bark and splintery in the wood.

Odour : Faint and characteristic.

Taste : Sweet.

CHEMICAL TESTS

A thick section or powder of the drug when treated with 80% sulphuric acid, gives orange yellow colour. It is due to the change of flavone glycoside to chalcone glycoside.

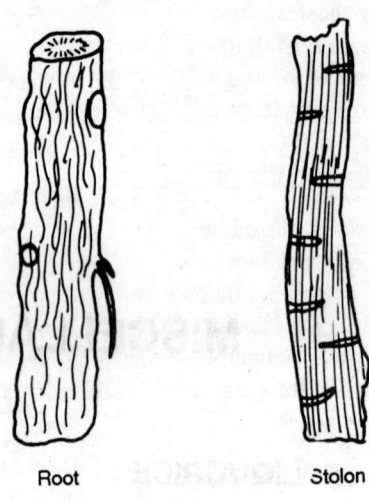

Root   Stolon

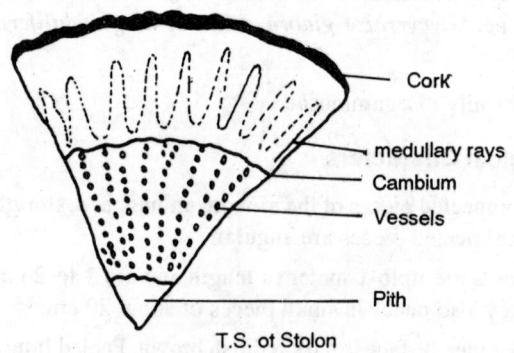

Cork

medullary rays

Cambium

Vessels

Pith

T.S. of Stolon

Fig. 36. Liquorice root

2. GARLIC

Garlic is a dried ripe bulb of *Allium sativum,* Linn

Family : Liliaceae

CHARACTERS

Form : Garlic occurs as a subglobular compound bulb.

Size : 4-6 cm in diameter with several (8-20) cloves.

Outer surface : The whole bulb is surrounded by 3-5 whitish papery membranous scales from the leaf bases of the previous years bulb and terminating in a thick, papery outgrowth. The cloves are attached to a flattened circular woody axis with numerous thin, wiry roots on the underside and short, subcylindrical outgrowth on the upper surface.

CHARACTERS OF THE CLOVE OF GARLIC

Each clove is ovoid, 3-5 sided, surrounded by two papery scale leaves, the outer one whitish and loose and inner one pink and adherent but easily separable from the solid portion of the clove. These papery scale leaves enclose two whitish, fleshy scales, the inner one thinner and smaller than the outer one. Two yellowish green, conduplicate (right half of the leaf is folded upon the left half length wise) foliage leaves present in the centre.

Odour : Strongly alliaceous

Taste : Persistently pungent, alliaceous

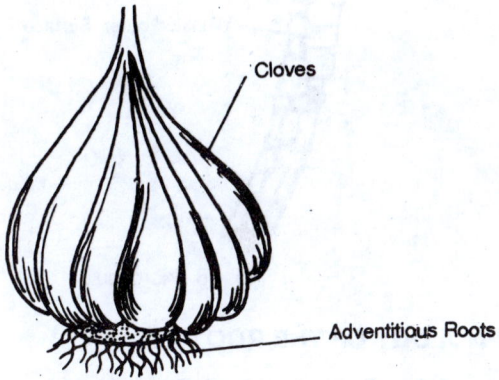

Fig. 37. Garlic

3. PICRORHIZA

It consist of dried roots and rhizomes of *Picrorhiza kurroa*. **Royale ex Benth.**

Family : Scrophulariaceae

MORPHOLOGCAL CHARACERS

From : The rhizome is cylindrical in shape.

SIze : 3-6 cm. long and 0.5-1 cm broad.

Outer surface : Outer surface shows closely set scale leaves which are present on the younger part of rhizome and on the older part scars of scale leaves encircling the upper half of circumferance. Conical bud and rhamnents of scar of stems are also present.

Colour : It is deep greenish brown.

Odour : Slightly unpleasant

Some loose roots are also present in the drug.

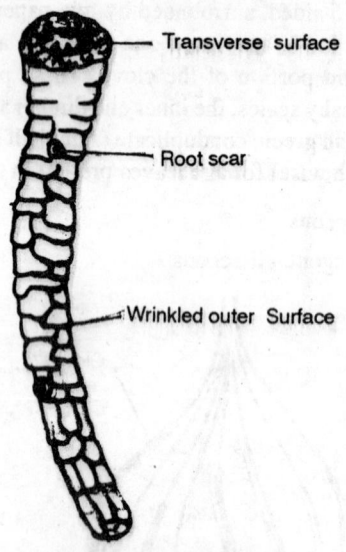

Fig. 38. Picrorhiza

MORPHOLOGY OF THE ROOT

Colour and size : Roots are about 1 mm. in diameter and dark grey in colour.

Shape : Straight or slightly curved.

Outer Surface : It is longitudinally wrinkled.

Fracture : Short.

Fractured Surfrace : A thin brown cork and black lacunous bark is seen. A circle of 5 pale tangentially extended. Xylem bundles with central pith are seen.

4. DIOSCOREA

Discorea consists of the tubers of several species of Dioscerea like *D. deltoidea* Wall., *D. prazeri* Prain, *D. floribunda* Mart and *D. Composita*.

Family : Dioscoreaceae

MORPHOLOGY

Tubers of variable size and shape are born on the stems. In some species cylindrical tubers penetrating deep into the ground are produced while in some species glabose tubers of large size are produced. They may be solitary or clustured together at the base of plant.

5. LINSEED

Linseed is the dried ripe seed of *Linum usitatissimum* Linn. belonging to family Linaceae.

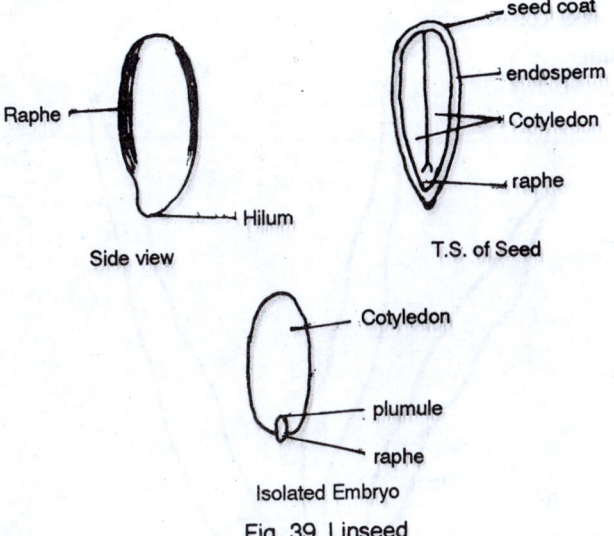

Fig. 39. Linseed

MORPHOLOGICAL CHARACTERS OF SEED

Shape : The seeds are elongated avoid and strongly flattend. It is rounded at one end and pointed at the other.

Size : 4-6 mm. long, 2-3 mm. wide and 1.5 mm thick.

Outer surface : The proximal end of the seed is pointed. Hilum is in a slight hollow on the more acute edge close to the pointed end. The raphe extends as a yellowish line along the quite edge from the hilum to other round end of seed.

Colour : Surface is brown and glossy.

Odour : None.

Taste : Mucilageneous and oily.

6. SHATAVARI

The drug consists of dried tuberous roots of *Asparagus racemosus* wild.

Family : Liliaceae

CHARACTERS

Shape : The roots are cylindrical, fleshy tuberous, tapering towards the base and swollen in the middle.

Size : 5-15 cm in length and 1-2 cm in diameter.

Colour : It is white to buff coloured. When it is soaked in water, it becomes soft and swells considerably.

Taste : Bitter.

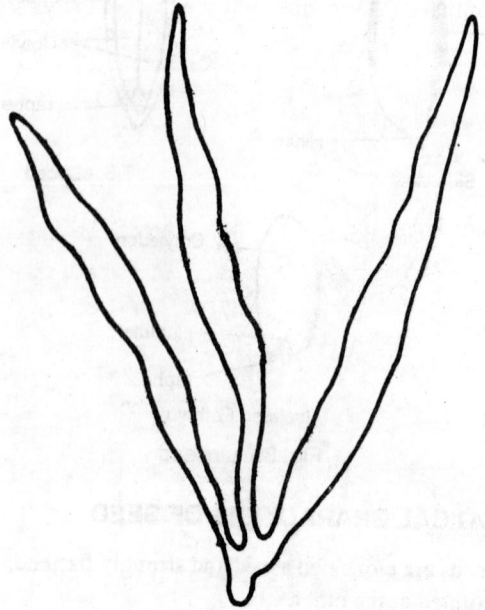

Fig 40 Shatavari

7. SHANKHPUSHPI

The drug consists of whole dried herb of *Convolvulus pluricaulis* (Syn : *Convolvulus microphyllus*) and *Evolvulus alsinoides* L.

Family : Convolvulaceae

CHARACTERS OF *C. PLURICAULIS*

The plant is a procumbent herb.

Stem : Woody at the base.

Leaves : The leaves are linear, elliptical subsessile having trichomes on both the surfaces.

Flowers : The flowers are short, axillary, solitary or 2-3 together, rose coloured or white.

CHARACTERS OF *E. ALSINOIDES*

This plant is a hairy perenial herb with prostrate branches arising from a small woody rootstock. The leaves are simple, sessile, alternate, lanceolate to suborbicular. Solitary flowers are light blue and the fruit is a four angled capsule.

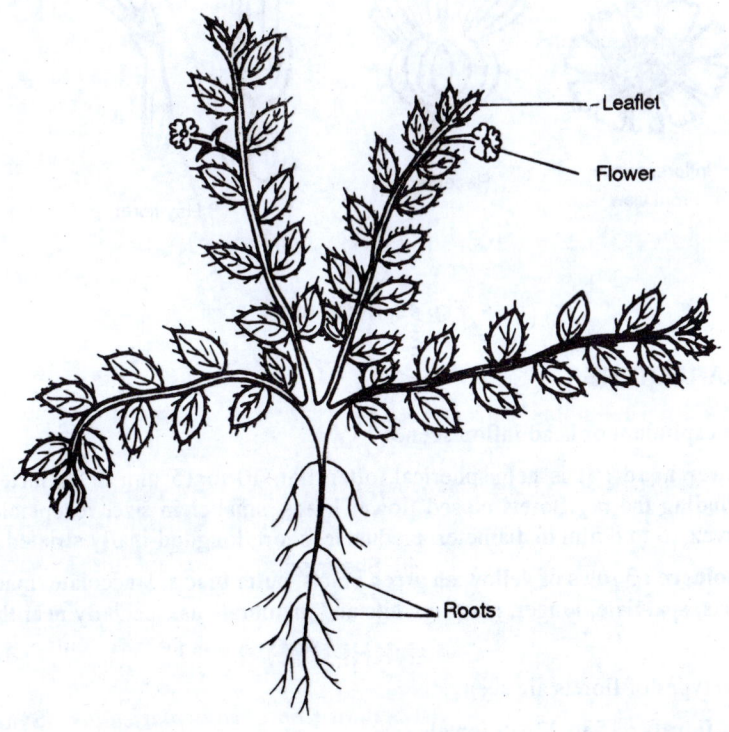

Fig. 41. Shankhpushpi

8. PYRETHRUM

Pyrethrum consists of the dried, closed or half open flowers of *Chrysanthemum cinerariifolium* Vis.

Family : Compositae

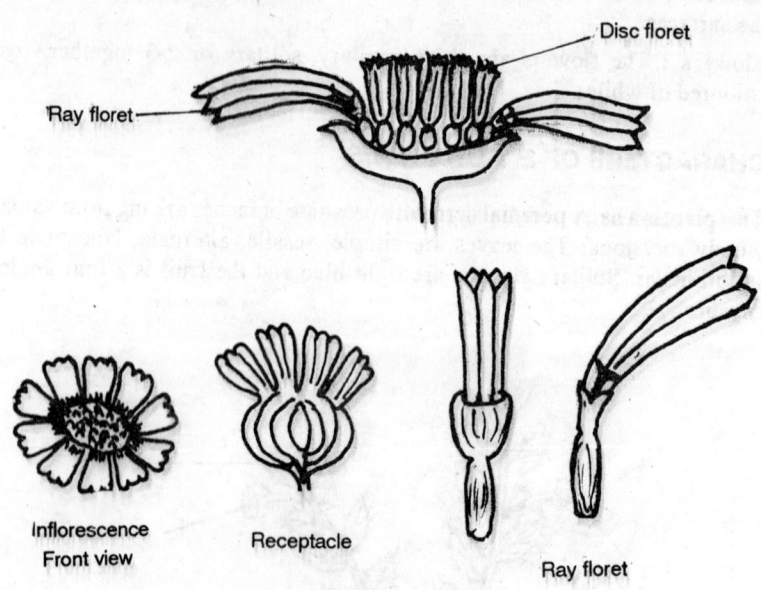

Fig. 42. Pyrethrum

CHARACTERS

It is capitulum or head inflorescence

Flower head : It is hemispherical, often flat, 10 to 15 mm in diameter. excluding the ray florets closed flower heads, smaller in size, receptacle, convex, 5 to 8 mm in diameter, preduncle, short, longitud-inally striated.

Involucre : 3 rows of yellowish green bracts, outer bracts, lanceolate, inner bracts, spatulate, longer, margin white and membranous, specially near the tip.

Two types of florets are seen

Ray florets : 15 to 23, all female.

Corolla : Cream or straw coloured, ligulate, oblong, shrivelled, 15 to 20 mm long, 15 to 17 veined, 3 small rounded teeth at the apex, central one smallest

Disc floret : 200 to 300 hermaphrodite, each having a yellow tubular corolla with 5 short lobes at the submit.

Fruit : Cypsela, 5 ribbed, oblong, about 5 mm long, surrounded by a membranous tubular calyx about 1 mm long.

Odour : Faint but characteristic

Taste : Bitter

9. TOBACCO

Tobacco consist of leaves and herb of *Nicotiana tabacum* Linn.

Family : Solanaceae

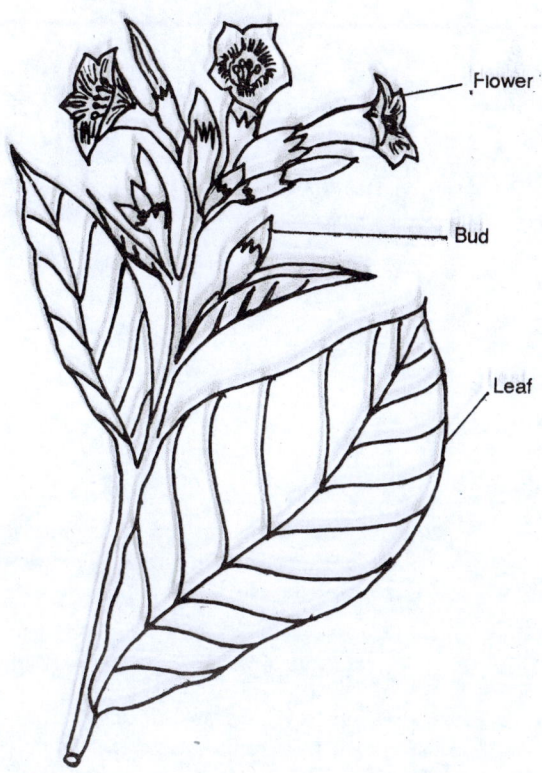

Fig. 43. Tobacco

MORPHOLOGICAL CHARACTERS OF PLANT

Plant is a tall annual herb stem is simple

Leaves : Ovate in shape with pubescent surface.

Margin : Entire

Base : Decurrent

Flowers : Long, tubular, pink or reddish and occur in terminal spreading cymes.

Odour : Characteristic

Taste : Characteristic bitter

23

FIBRES

1. COTTON

Cotton is the epidermal hairs of the seeds of cultivated species of *Gossypium herbaceum*.

> Family : Malvaceae

Absorbent cotton is prepared from the raw cotton by removing fatty material and other impurities and then bleached and sterilized.

CHARACTERS OF ABSORBENT COTTON

Absorbent cotton is a pure form of cellulose which occurs in the form of thin fine filament like hairs. The trichomes are unicellular 2-4 cm in length and 25-40 μ in diameter. It is a loosely felted mass of delicate filament, soft to touch and white in colour. Raw cotton has slight brown tint, a colour which is due to the dried remains of protoplasm and cell contents, the wall of the trichomes being quite transparent and colourless. Absorbent cotton rapidly sinks when placed on water, the non absorbent or raw cotton floats due to the presence of fatty material in the cuticle.

CHEMICAL TESTS

(i) Mount few fibres in cuoxam (A freshly prepared ammonical copper oxide solution). Examine under microscope. Raw cotton shows granular cuticle and uneven swelling; ballooning in cuoxan. Absorbent cotton show uniform swelling and final solution in cuoxam.

(ii) Cotton fibre is soluble in 80% w/w sulphuric acid but insoluble in 60% acid.

(iii) It is insoluble in concentrated hydrochloric acid.

(iv) Moister the fibre with iodine (N/50) followed by a drop of 8% w/w sulphuric acid, a blue colour is produced.

(v) Warm with Millon's reagent, no red stain. (distinction from wool and silk).

(vi) On ignition, cotton fibres burn with flame but no foul smell. It leaves white ash.

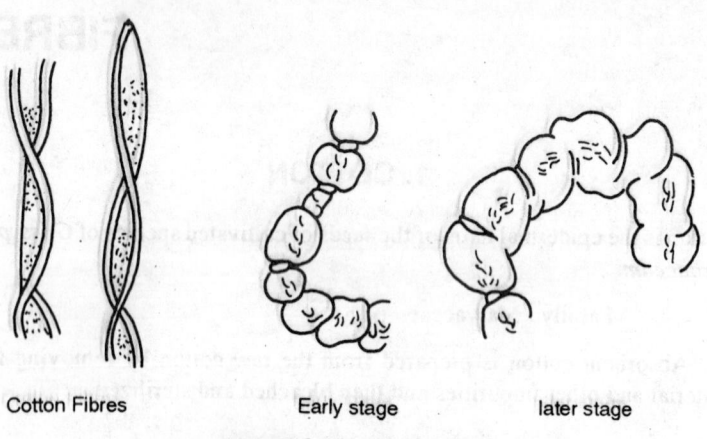

Cotton Fibres	Early stage	later stage

(after treatment with cuaxam)

Fig. 44 (a) Swelling in cuaxam

2. SILK

Silk is a fibre made from the cocoons of *Bombyx mori* Linn.

Family : Bombycidae

Which feed on the leaves of mulberry plant, *Morus alba* Linn.

Family : Moraceae

Silk is also obtained from the larvae of *Anthoroea* species.

Family : Saturnidae

CHARACTERS

Silk fibres are very fine, smooth and solid and are usually yellow in colour. Silk is soft and smooth to the touch, possesses considerable tensile strength and elasticity and is hygroscopic.

CHEMICAL TESTS

(i) In cuoxam solution, it is partially soluble.

(ii) In 80% and 60% w/w sulphuric acid, it is soluble.

(iii) In 50% potassium hydroxide solution, it is soluble.

(iv) In concentrated hydrochloric acid, it is rapidly soluble.

(v) With N/50 iodine solution followed by 8% sulphuric acid, it gives yellow colour.

(vi) Warm or boil in a test tube with picric acid solution, permanent yellow colour is produced.

(vii) Warm with Millon's reagent, it gives red stain.

(vii) Warm with 5% potassium hydroxide solution. Then add lead acetate solution. White precipitate is produced.

(viii) On ignition, brown gases which are alkaline to litmus are produced. There is foul smell (like burnt hair or flesh). It burns slowly giving beads followed by white ash.

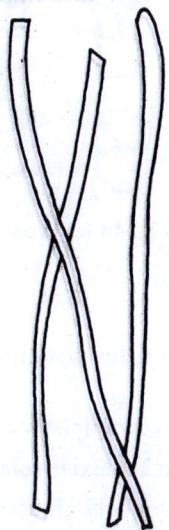

Fig. 44 (b) Silk fibre

3. WOOL

Wool consists of the hairs from the fleeces of the sheep, *Ovis aries* Linn.

Family : Bovidae

der : Ungulata

CHARACTERS

Wool occurs as a loosely felted mass of elastic, lustrous, more or less curly hairs, smooth and somewhat slippery to touch. It is hygroscopic and absorb about 50 to 60 percent moisture. A wad of wool resists tearing with considerable force, owing to the tendency of the hairs to cling together.

Wool consists of more or less curved, subcylindrical threads, covered with irregular lines crossing them transversely at fairly close intervals and connected by other lines at right angles to them. A dark coloured narrow band is present along the central axis of many of the hairs and is called medulla. The fibres are about 15 to 25 or 45 to 60 µ in width. Wool fibre polarise brightly with crossed nicols, many hair show bright colour.

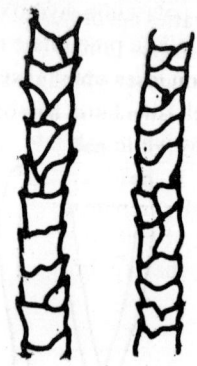

Fig. 44 (c) Wool fibre

CHEMICAL TEST

(i) In cuoxam solution, the wool fibres are insoluble but swell and scales separate.

(ii) In 80% and 60% w/w sulphuric acid, it is insoluble.

(iii) In 50% potassium hydroxide solution, it is insoluble.

(iv) In concentrated hydrochloric acid, it is insoluble.

(v) Moisten the wool fibres with N/50 iodine solution followed by a drop of 8% w/w sulphuric acid, a yellow colour is produced.

(vi) Warm/boil the fibres with picric acid. Then rinse well with water, permanent yellow stain is produced.

(vii) Warm with Millon's reagent, red stain is produced.

(vii) Warm with 5% potassium hydroxide solution. Then add lead acetate solution, black precipitate is produced.

(ix) On ignition, brown gases which are alkaline to litmus are produced. The gas has foul odour (like burnt of hair or flesh). It burns slowly giving beads followed by white ash.

REGENERATED FIBRES
4. VISCOSE RAYON

Viscose rayon is a prepared fibre made from purified cellulose. The cellulose is obtained from various coniferous wood.

CHARACTERS

Viscose rayon fibres are white and lustrous fibres. They have refractive index of 1.53. The tensile strength varies according to the finish treatment to which it is subjected and may be from two thirds to one and half times more that of cotton. When wetted, the rayon loses upto 60 per cent of its tensile strength.

The fibres are solid and transparent having a diameter of about 15 μ to 25 μ. They are marked by longitudinal lines, which correspond to grooves in the surface of the fibres. In transverse sections the grooves appear as indentation and give an irregular crenate margin. The fibres are clearly visible in lactophenol or in solution of chloral hydrate, but are almost invisible in cresol, in all these mountants they are brilliantly luminous in polarized light with crossed micols.

CHEMICAL TESTS

(i) In cuoxam solution, it is soluble with uniform swelling.

(ii) It is soluble in 80% at 60% w/w sulphuric acid solution.

(iii) In 5% potassium hydroxide, it is insoluble but acquires yellow tint.

(iv) In concentrated hydrochloric acid it is insoluble.

(v) Moisten with N/50 iodine followed by a drop of 8% w/w sulphuric acid, a blue colour is produced.

(vi) Warm/boil in a test tube with picric acid solution and then rinse with water, No permanent yellow stain is produced.

(vii) Warm with Millon's reagent, no red stain is produced.

(viii) On ignition, it burns with flame but no foul odour is produced. Also there is no bead formation. It leaves white ash.

5. ACETATE RAYON

Acetate rayon is partially acetylated cellulose prepared from cotton fibres or wood cellulose.

CHARACTERS

The acetate rayon filaments are highly lustrous, grooved and slightly twisted. It is very much like viscose rayon and hence resemble very much with it.

6. ALGINATE YARN

Alginate rayon is composed of calcium alginate precipitated as continuous filaments.

CHARACTERS

The alginate fibres are cream coloured lustrous filaments. The layer filaments may be reduced to staple size which may be processed to calcium alginate wool or converted into gauze. Alginate fibres may also be processed into absorbable haemostatic dressings. These are soluble in 5 per cent sodium citrate solution.

CHEMICAL TESTS OF CALCIUM ALGINATE

   (i) In cuoxam solution, it is soluble with uniform swelling.

  (ii) In 80% w/w sulphuric acid solution it is soluble with swelling.

 (iii) In 60% w/w sulphuric acid solution, it is insoluble.

  (iv) In 5% potassium hydroxide solution, it is insoluble but acquires yellow tint.

   (v) In concentrated hydrochloric acid, it is insoluble.

  (vi) In 5% sodium citrate solution, it is soluble.

 (vii) Moisten wilt N/50 iodine solution, followed by a drop of 8% w/w sulphuric acid, no blue colour is produced instead brown red colour is produced.

(viii) Warm or boil with picric acid, and rinse with water, no permanent yellow colour is produced.

  (ix) Warm with Million's reagent, no red stain is produced.

Table.

Common Name	Synonym	Official Source	Category of Active Constituents	Important Active Constituents	Uses
CHAPTER-2					
Aloe	Musabbar	Aloe species Liliaceae	Anthraquinone glycosides	Aloin, (barbaloin) β-barbaloin,	Internally as purgative Externally in skin diseases
Rhubarb	Rheum	*Rheum* Species Polygonaceae	-do-	Free anthraquinones	purgative
Caster oil	Oleum Ricini	*Ricinus communis* Euphorbiaceae	Triglycerides of fatty acids	Triglycerides of ricinoleic, Isoricinoleic acid	Internally as cathartic Externally as emollient
Ispaghula	Ishabgul	*Plantago ovata* Plantaginaceae	Hydrocolloid Polysaccharide	Polysaccharide yeilds L-arabiose, rhamnose D-galactose and D-galacturonic acid.	Bulk laxative in chronic constipation
Senna	Tinnevelly Senna Alexanderian Senna	*Cassia angustifolia Cassia acutifolia* Leguminosae	Anthraquinone glycosides	Sennoside A, Sennoside B, Sennoside C, Sennoside D, Aloe emodin, Chrysophanol	laxative;
CHAPTER-3					
Digitalis	Foxglove leaves	*Digitalis purpurea* Scrophulariaceae	Cardiac glycosides	Primary glycosides are purpurea glycoside A & B secondary glycosides are digitoxin, gitoxin and digoxin	congestive cardiac failure Atrial flutter Atrial fibrillation
Arjuna Bark	Arjuna	*Terminalia arjuna* Combretaceae	Saponins tannins	Triterpenoidal saponins tannins	Diuretic to decrease blood pressure and heart rate.

Table

Common Name	Synonym	Official Source	Category of Active Constituents	Important Active Constituents	Uses
CHAPTER-4					
Coriander	Coriandrum	*Coriandrum sativum* Umbelliferae	Volatile oil	Coriandrol (linalool), pinene, geraniol, borneol	Flavouring agent, carminative, spice
Fennel	Foeniculum	*Foeniculum vulgare* Umbelliferae	-do-	Chief constituents thymol	Carminative, Flavouring agent
Ajowan	Ajwian	*Trachyspermum ammi* Umbelliferae	-do-	Volatile oil contains thymol	Carminative, spice
Cardamom	Cardamoni fructus	*Elettaria cardamomum* var. minuscula Zingiberaceae	-do-	It contains cineole and terpinyl acetate	Carminative, flavouring agent
Ginger	Ginger	*Zingiber officinale* Zingiberaceae	Volatile oil	Volatile oil contains zaingiberene, zingiberol	Stimulant, carminative flavouring agent
Black pepper	Pepper	*Piper nigram* Piperaceae	-do-	It contains terpenes β-pinene and phellanerene	Internally as stimulant
Asafoetida Nutmeg	Myristica	*Myristica fragrans* Myristicaceae	-do-	myristicin, elemicin	Carminative, Externally in rheumatism
Cinnamon	Cinnamon	*Cinnamomum zeylanicum* Lauraceae	-do- Tannins	It contains cinnamic aldehyde and eugenol Phlobatannins	Carminative, flavouring agent, Astringent
Clove	Caryophyllum	*Eugenia caryophyllus* Myrtaceae	Volatile oil	It contains eugenol vanillin	Carminative flavouring agent antiseptic dental pain

Table **125**

Table

Common Name	Synonym	Official Source	Category of Active Constituents	Important Active Constituents	Uses
CHAPTER-5					
Catechu Black catechu	Catechu Nigrum	*Acacia catechu* Leguminosae	Tannins	Catechin, catechutannic acid	Astringent, in diarrhoea
Pale catechu	Gambier catechu	*Uncaria gambier* Rubiaceae	Tannins	Catechin, catechutannic and Gambier fluorescin	Bleeding of gums
CHAPTER-6					
Hyoscymus	henbane	*Hyoscymus niger* solanaceae	tropane alkaloids	Hyoscyamine and traces hyoscine	Cerebral and spinal sedative
Belladonna	Deadly nightshade	*Atropa belladonna* Solanaceae	-do-	Hyoscyamine Hyoscine, atropine	Respiratory sedative. Spasmodytic cough, Externally as local anaethetic
Aconite	Radix Aconiti	*Aconitum napellus* Renunculaceae	Alkaloids	Aconitine, picraconitine, aconine, mesaconitine hypaconitine and neopalline	Neuralgia, rheumatism (externally)
Ephedra	Ma haung	Ephedra spp. Gnetaceae	-do-	Ephderine, psendoephedrine N-methyl ephedrine and Nor-d-ephedrine	Acts on C.N.S. as sympathomimetic
Opium	Opium	*Papaver somniferum* Papaveracea	-do-	25 alkaloids morphine, codeine, thebaine, papaverine, narcotine	Hypnotic, sedative habit forming so not used now a days.

Table.

Common Name	Synonym	Official Source	Category of Active Constituents	Important Active Constituents	Uses.
Cannabis	Indian Hemp	*Canabis sativa* Cannabinaceae	Resin	Tetrahydrocannabinol Cannabinol, Cannobigerol, Cannabidiol, Cannabidiolic acid	Sedative, in hysteria, spasmodic cough Habit forming so not used now a days
Nux-vomica	Semina strychni	*Strychnos nuxvomica* Loeganiaceae	Alkaloids	Strychnine, Brucine	Bitter stomachic. Excites the motor nerves lead to convulsions
CHAPTER - 7					
Raulwolfia	Indian snake Root	*Rauwolfia serpentina* Apocyanaceae	Alkaloids	Reserpine Ajmaline, ajamalicine, serpen tinine	Psychotic disorders and as anti hypertensive Traquillizer
CHAPTER - 8					
Vasaka	Adhatoda	*Adhatoda vasica* Acanthaceae	alkaloids	Vasicine Vasicinone	Vasicine is abortifacient Vasicinene is broncho-dilator
Tolu Balsam	Balsamum Tolutanum	*Myroxylon balsamum* Leguminosae	Resin esters	Toluresinotannol cinnamate and benzoate, benzyl cinnamate, bezoic acid, cinnamic acid, vanillin etc.	Expectorant flavouring agent in medicinal syrups
Tulsi	Sacred basil	*Ocimum sanctum* Labiatae	Volalite oil	Eugenol, methyl euginol caryophyllin	Expectorant, aromatic, carminative antibacterial, antiprotozoal

Table **127**

Table

Common Name	Synonym	Official Source	Category of Active Constituents	Important Active Constituents	Uses
CHAPTER - 9					
Colchicum	Colchici cormus	*Colchicum autumnale* Liliaceae	Alkaloids	Colchicine Demecolcine	pain and inflammation of acute gout, colchicine is tumour inhibitory in nature
Guggal	Balsamoderdron Mukul	*Commiphora mukul* Burseraceae	Oleogum resin	Important constituents are 2-guggulsterone, guggulsterol I & II,III	Anti-in flammatory, Hypo-lipidimic Now a days tried in diabetes and Hypertension
CHAPTER 10					
Vinca	Catharanthus	*Catharanthus roseus* Apocyanaceae	Alkaloid	Vincristine, Vinb-lastine, Ajmalicine serpentine	Hodgkin's disease. Chorio-carcinoma, in Leukemia
CHAPTER 11					
Chaulmooga oil	Hydnocarpus oil	*Hydnocarpus wightiana* Flacourtiaceae	Oil	Oil contains acids like Hydnocarpic acid, chaulmoogric acid	Antileprotic
CHAPTER 12					
Pterocarpus	Kino vijayasar	*Pterocarpus marsu pium* Leguminosae	Flavones	Liquiritigenin Isoliquiritigenin marsupol	Hypoglycemic agent in diabetes, gum is useful in dysentery

Table

Common Name	Synonym	Official Source	Category of Active Constituents	Important Active Constituents	Uses
Gymnema sylvestre	Gurmar	*Gymnema sylvestre* Asclepiadaceae	Acid	Gymnemic acid	In Diabetes. In Ayurveda as stomachic, stimulant
CHAPTER - 13					
Gokhru	Chota Gokhru	*Tribulus terrestris* Zygophyllaceae	Saponins	Saponins on hydro-lysis yeilds dios-genin, gitogenin ruscogenin	Drug is diuretic so useful in nephritis and kidney stone gout and painful micturition
	Bara Gokhru	*Pedalium murex* Pedaliaceae	Fatty oil, resin, mucilage	Fatty oil	
Punarnava	Hogweed	*Boerhaavia diffusa* Nyctaginaceae	Alkaloids acids	Punarnavine urolic acid stearic acid	Diuretic, Anti in flammatory
CHAPTER - 14					
Ipecacuanha	Ipecac	*Cephailis ipecacuanha* Rubiaceae	Alkaloids Glycoside	Emetine, cephaeline, psychotrine, Ipecoside	Amoebic dysentery, Expectorant,
CHAPTER- 15					
Benzoin	Gum Benjamin	*Styrax benzoin* Styraceae	Balsamic acids	Free balsamic acids like cinnamic acid, benzoic acid	Antiseptic, Disinfectant, Expectorant

Table **129**

Table

Common Name	Synonym	Official Source	Category of Active Constituents	Important Active Constituents	Uses
			Triterpenoid acids siaresinolic acid	Sumaresinolic acid	Antiseptic, Disinfectant, mouth wash
Myrrh	Myrrha	*Commiphora molmol* Burseraceae	oleogum resin	Oil contains terpenes ester, cuminic aldehyde Resin contains α, β and γ-commiphoric acids.	
Nim	Neem	*Azadirachta indica* Meliaceae	Neem oil	Azadirachtin Azadirinin Azadirone	Bitter tonic, astringent Skin diseases Insectiside, pesticide
Curcuma	Indian saffron	*Curcuma longa* Zingiberaceae	Colouring matter volatile oil	curcumins like curcumin I,II & III Volatile lil contains tumerone and zingi-berene	Colouring agent, Antiseptic Anti-inflammatory
CHAPTER - 16					
Chinchona	Peruvian Bark	Cinchona species Rubiaceae	Alkaloids	Quinine, quinidine, Cinchonine	Antimalarial, Bitter tonic, Stomachic
CHAPTER - 17					
Ergot	Rye ergot	*Claviceps purpurea* clavicipitaceae	-do-	Water soluble ergometrine type. Water insoluble ergotoxine type of alkoloids	Oxytocic to stimulate uterine muscles to induce delivery

Table

Common Name	Synonym	Official Source	Category of Active Constituents	Important Active Constituents	Uses
CHAPTER - 18					
Shark liver oil	Oleum Selachide	Liver of fish Hypoprion brevirostris (braevirodstris)	Vitamine rich oil	Oil contains vitamin A and glycerides of saturated and unsaturated fatty acids.	Nutritive and tonic, Xerophthalmia
Amla	Embelica	*Embelica officinalis* Euphorbiaceae	Vitamin	Vitamin C	Scurvy, Antifungal, Anti viral
CHAPTER - 19					
Papaya	Papita	*Carica papaya* Caricaceae	Enzyme	Papain	Proteolytic enzyme
Diastase	Diastase	Barley grains Graminae	-do-	Diastase	Starch digesting enzyme
Yeast	Yeast	*Saccharmyces cerevisae* Saccharomycetaceae	Vitamins	B-group vitamins namely Aneurine, Riboflavine, Nicotine, Pyridoxine, Pentothenic Acid	Vitamin supplement
			Engyme	Zymase, maltase,	
Asafoetida	Asafetida	*Ferula foetida* Umbelleferae	Oleagum resin	Oil contains organic disulphide Resin contais asaresinol ferulate, free ferulic acid	Antispasmodic laxative

Table 131

Table

Common Name	Synonym	Official Source	Category of Active Constituents	Important Active Constituents	Uses
CHAPTER - 20					
Peppermint oil	Mentha Piperita oil	*Mentha piperita* Labiatae	Volatile oil	It contains free menthol, menthofuran, jasmone, esters of menthol, piperine, Piperitone	Flavouring agent in perfumey, aromatic, carminative counter-irritant, carmative
Lemon oil	Oil limonis	*Citrus limon* Rutaceae	volatile oil	Oil contains citral, geranyl and linanyl acetate	Aromatic, carminative, flavouring agent
Orange oil	Oil aurantia	*Citrus sinensis* Rutaceae	Volatile oil	Oil contains limonine elixits	Flavouring agent in aromatic
Lemon grass Oil	Indian melissa	*Cymbopogan citratus* Graminae	-do-	Oil contains Terpene aldenyde citral	α-Inones is made form citral is important flavouring agent.
Sandal wood	Sandal wood	*Santalum album* Santalaceae	-do-	Oil contains free alcohols, α and β santols, α and β santalenes, santalone and santenone	Used in cosmetics, perfumery, medicinally as stimulat
CHAPTER - 21					
Honey	Madhu	*Apis indica* Apidae	Carbohydrate	Invert sugar, enzymes	Pharmaceutical aid Demulscent, laxative
Arachis oil	Peanut oil	*Arachis hypogea*	Lipids	Glycerides of oleic	Pharmaceutical aid,

Table

Common Name	Synonym	Official Source	Category of Active Constituents	Important Active Constituents	Uses
		Leguminosae		linoleic, palmitic, strearic, Arichidic, Lignoceric acid	solvent in injections
Starch	Amylum Maize Starch Rice starch Wheat Starch	Zea mays Oryza sativa Triticum aestivum Graminae	Carbohydrate	Polysaccharide water soluble part is amylose	Nutritive, protective, Demulscent
	Potato Starch	Solanum tuberosum Solanaceae		Water in soluble part is amylopectin	
Kaolin	China clay	Clay	Mineral	Aluminium Silicate with traces of magnesium calcium, iron	Light kaolin in G.I.T. infection, Heavy Kaolin as excipient in poultice
Pectin	Pectin	Different fruits like lemon, orange, apple Guava	Pectin polymer	It gives pectinic acids which are derivatives of galacturonic acids	In diarrhoea. As thickening agent
Olive	Olum olivae	Olea europoea Olaceae	Lipids	Oil contains oleic acid, linoleic acid, palmitic and stearic acid	Pharmaceutical aid in the preparation of cosmetics, soaps etc.
Lanoin	Hydrous wool	Ovis aries Bovidae	Lipids	Esters of Lanoceric, Carnaubic, myristic acid	Pharmaceutical aid, Emollient base for creams and ointments.
Bees wax	Bees wax	Apis mellifera	Wax	Wax contains myricyl	Used in the preparation of

Table **133**

Table

Common Name	Synonym	Official Source	Category of Active Constituents	Important Active Constituents	Uses
		Apidae		acetate and free wax acids like cerotic acids	ointments, plasters
Acacia	Babul	*Acacia senegal* Leguminosae	Carbohy-drate	It consist of arabin which is mixture of calcium, magnesium and potassium salt of arabic acid	Emulsifying agent, Binding Agent Suspending agent, Demulscent
Tragacanth	Gum tragacanth	*Astragalus gummifer* Leguminosae	Carbohydrate	Water soluble portion is tragacanthin and water insoluble portion is bassorin	Laxative, Demulscent, sus-pending agent, emulsifying agent
Sodium alginate	Alginate	Lamineria species Laminariaceae	Carbohydrate	Sodium salt of alginic acid	Phrmaceutical aid, adhe-sive, Emulsifying agent
Agar	Agar-Agar	Geladium species Gelidiaceae	Corbohydrate Polycaccharide	Polysaccharide consists of agarose agaropectin	Bulk laxative, suspending agent, Emulsifier, Nutrient medium
Guargum	Guaran	*Cyamopsis Tetragonolobus* Leguminosae	Gum	Hydro colloidal Polysac-charide which gives gal-actose and mannose on hydrolysis	Thickenning agent. Emul-stifing agent, Bulk laxative. In diabetes
Gelatin	Gelatin	Collagen from skin bones and conective tissues of animals	Protein	It contains glutin which is made up of 18 different amino acids.	Pharmaceutical aid in hard and soft gelatin capsules and also in cosmetic industry.

Table

Common Name	Synonym	Official Source	Category of Active Constituents	Important Active Constituents	Uses
CHAPTER - 22					
Liquorice	Glycyrrhiza	*Glycyrrhiza glabra* Leguminosae	Glycosides Flavonoids	Glycyrrhizin which yeilds glycyrrhetinic acid It also contains chalcone glycoside isoliquiritin	Epectorant, demulscent, laxative, Antipeptic ulcer
Garlic	Lehsun	*Allium sativum* Liliaceae	Essential oil	It contains allicin allin and a polysulphide	Antibacterial, G.I.T. stimulant
Picrorhiza	Kutki	*Picrorhiza kurroa* Scrophulariaceae	Glycosides	Iridoid type of glycosides consist of picrorrhizin Picroride A and Kutkoside	Bitter tonic, liver disorders, In jaundice.
Diescorea steridal	yams	*Dioscorea deltoida* Dioscoreaceae	Saponin glycoside	Diosgenin mainly Traces of heccogenin	precursor for making steroidal drugs. In Ayurveda as fish and lice poision.
Linseed	Flax seed	*Linum usitatissimum* Linaceae	Fixed oil Glycoside mucilage	Oil contains unsatrurated acids cyanogenetic glycoside, linamarin	Demulscent, laxative. Externally in poultice
Shatavari	Satavari	*Asparagus racemosus* Liliaceae	Saponin glycosides	Saponin A4, A5, A6 and A8. Sarasapo-genin from hydrolysis of A4 saponin	Diuretic, Aphrodiasic, Nutritive, tonic
Shankhu-	Shankhapushp	*Evolvulus alsinoides*	Alkaloids	Betain,	Bitter tonic, anthelmintic,

Table **135**

Table—

Common Name	Synonym	Official Source	Category of Active Constituents	Important Active Constituents	Uses
pushpi		Convolvulaceae		Evolvine	Nervine tonic, nervous debility
Pyrethrum	Insect Flower	*Chrysanthemum cinerarifolium* Compositae	Esters	Terpenes Cinerin I,II Jasmolin I,II	Pyrethrin I,II Insectiside against flies, insects, mosquitoes
Tobacco	Tambaku	*Nicotiana tabacum* Solanaceae	Alkaloids	Nicotine, Nor-nicotine Anabasine, Nicoteine	Insectiscide, fish poison Narcotic, Sedative, emetic

INDEX